Understanding Multiple Sclerosis

Understanding Health and Sickness Series
Miriam Bloom, Ph.D.
General Editor

Understanding Multiple Sclerosis

Melissa Stauffer, Ph.D.

University Press of Mississippi
Jackson

www.upress.state.ms.us

The University Press of Mississippi is a member of the Association of American University Presses.

Copyright © 2006 by University Press of Mississippi
All rights reserved
Manufactured in the United States of America

First edition 2006

Illustrations by Alan Estridge

Library of Congress Cataloging-in-Publication Data

Stauffer, Melissa.
    Understanding multiple sclerosis / Melissa Stauffer.
        p. ; cm. — (Understanding health and sickness series)
    Includes bibliographical references and index.
    ISBN 1-57806-802-9 (cloth : alk. paper) — ISBN 1-57806-803-7
(pbk. : alk. paper) 1. Multiple sclerosis—Popular works.
    [DNLM: 1. Multiple Sclerosis, Chronic Progressive—diagnosis—
Popular Works. 2. Multiple Sclerosis, Chronic Progressive—therapy—
Popular Works. WL 360 S798u 2006] I. Title. II. Understanding
health and sickness series.
    RC377.S73   2006
    616.8′34—dc22   2005018088

British Library Cataloging-in-Publication Data available

This book is affectionately dedicated to my sister, Heather, an MS survivor.

Contents

Acknowledgments

I thank my editor, Miriam Bloom, for her patience with this fledgling writer; my mother, Carolyn Pohl, for her suggestions for improving the glossary; and my scientific mentor, Walter Chazin, for recognizing my ability to write and encouraging me to do so. Special thanks go to Dr. Harold Moses, Jr., and Dr. John Bright, both of Vanderbilt University, for reviewing the manuscript and making valuable suggestions.

Introduction

Multiple sclerosis affects 2.5 million people worldwide and four hundred thousand Americans. It is the most common neurodegenerative disease in young adults, with a particularly high occurrence in women. In spite of erratic and variable symptoms, investigators have made great strides in diagnosing and treating MS during the last decade. This book, written for people who need to understand MS—those who have been recently diagnosed, their families and friends, or interested health care professionals—is intended to provide background on the history and biology of MS and to chronicle recent developments that allow people with MS today to live fuller and longer lives.

The book opens with a general introduction to the genetic, demographic, and geographic factors that correlate with MS incidence. The second chapter is devoted to the basic biology of MS, with descriptions of the central nervous system and the immune system and an explanation of their interaction during autoimmunity. The characteristic symptoms of MS are outlined in a discussion of the latest diagnostic criteria and the different types of MS. This is followed by a description of MS treatments, over-the-counter medications for specific symptoms, and alternative treatments with herbs and vitamins. Living with MS, including coping strategies, relational concerns, and long-term plans, is addressed in chapter 5. The book concludes with an overview of the current MS research that will impact the next generation of MS drugs.

Thanks to an ensemble of disease-modifying therapies, people with MS can live highly active lives. Inspirational examples include talk-show host Montel Williams, country singer Clay Walker, actress Teri Garr, and public policy-analyst Laura R. Mitchell. Many effective treatments are available, and the research outlook for MS is promising, with potential new drugs being discovered each year. It is my hope that this book will convince its readers that life with MS can be both positive and productive.

Understanding Multiple Sclerosis

1. Who Gets MS and Why?

Multiple sclerosis (MS) affects nearly 2.5 million people worldwide. About one in 750 Americans will be diagnosed with some form of the disease during their lifetime. Nearly 400,000 people in the United States have it right now, and two hundred new cases are diagnosed each week. Perhaps you know someone who has it.

The cause of MS is not known, but it has both genetic and environmental components. Scientists do not know exactly why certain people get MS, but clues to its underlying causes are found in studies of its prevalence—its rate of occurrence in families and across certain segments of the population. This chapter will introduce you to the genetic and environmental factors that are thought to play a role in causing MS and will discuss several interesting trends that provide insight into who gets MS and why.

Worldwide Distribution and Risk

Epidemiology is the study of the occurrence of a disease in relation to demographic, geographic, socioeconomic, and environmental variables. Epidemiologists who study MS have reported its incidence, prevalence, and associated mortality rates. Figure 1.1 shows these descriptors as a function of decade of life. The line for prevalence indicates that most people with MS are in their thirties or forties, with the average age of an MS patient being around forty-five. This reflects the usual delay between the first symptoms and the final diagnosis; MS

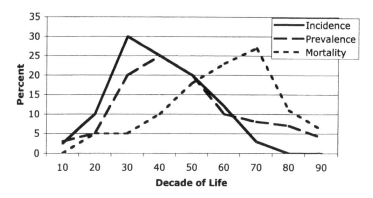

Figure 1.1 Rates of incidence, prevalence, and mortality for populations affected by MS. Incidence is the number of new diagnoses. Prevalence is the number of people who have been diagnosed at any given point in time. Mortality is the percentage of people who die directly from disease-related causes. The values reported correspond to the number of individuals per 100,000 people during one year. Reproduced from *McAlpine's Multiple Sclerosis*

symptoms typically appear in the twenties and early thirties, which is where the line for incidence peaks. MS patients can live into their early seventies or even longer, as shown by the line for mortality. The expected decrease in life span for a person with MS is only about five to seven years, equivalent to the results of smoking one pack of cigarettes per day. This long life span is largely due to the benefits of modern health care.

It is difficult to estimate accurately how many people have MS at any given time because of the delay between the onset of symptoms and the diagnosis. Accurate estimates of both incidence and mortality also depend on the age range of the people who make up the particular population being analyzed, so the numbers can vary from study to study. The average worldwide prevalence of MS is between 0.1 percent and 0.13 percent across all adult ages (twenty to ninety years of age). This means that 100 to 130 people have MS for every 100,000 in the population. A few comparisons may help put these numbers in perspective.

A recent study published in *Preventive Medicine* compared the risk of getting MS to the risk of getting other diseases such as cancer, diabetes, and Alzheimer disease. The lifetime risk estimates of getting MS were 0.25 percent for men and 0.36 percent for women. By comparison, the risk estimates for getting cancer were 38 percent for men and 30 percent for women. That means men and women are about 150 times and 83 times more likely to get cancer than MS, respectively.

The same study compared various causes of death, such as stroke, car accidents, and suicide, with the risk of dying from MS. The estimated risk of dying in a car accident, which is low relative to the risk of getting cancer or having a stroke but still represents a common cause of death, is 1.53 percent for men and 0.75 percent for women, two to six times the risks of getting MS.

Sex-linked Distribution

The above comparison of MS with cancer highlights one of the interesting epidemiological features of MS: that it is between two and three times more common in women than in men. The reason for this difference is not known. MS is only one of several autoimmune diseases more common in women, and the most likely explanation is that female hormones interact somehow with the immune system. Certain other disease characteristics are sex-related as well, including the average age at onset and the type of disease progression. The female:male ratio is highest for children, whereas in the fifth decade of life or later, men are more likely to be diagnosed. Men are also more likely to have an aggressive course of the disease.

Racial Distribution

Racial differences in incidence confirm a genetic component to MS. MS is most prevalent in people of northern European descent, although people from Africa, Asia, or South America are not immune. Because MS has historically been a disease of Caucasians, it has been most closely studied in Eastern Europe. To this day, Scotland reports the highest incidence rates of MS: 187 per 100,000. Tallies from Scandinavian countries (Norway, Sweden, Finland, Denmark, and Iceland) average about 100 per 100,000. Within Europe, differences in incidence correlate with ancestry. For instance, studies of Icelanders show that they are genetically distinct from their Norwegian neighbors in addition to having a comparatively lower incidence of MS. Similar genetic correlations have been observed in Italians, where the incidence is markedly higher in Sardinians than in those living on the mainland. Genetic isolation of these populations over centuries is the likely explanation for how these differences came to be. North American Caucasians have rates of MS of 50 to 100 per 100,000, though data from the western hemisphere is scant compared to those from Europe.

Many non-Caucasians have a remarkably low incidence of MS. These include black Africans, Mongolians, Chinese, Japanese, Native Americans, and Australian Aborigines. White Africans have a much higher incidence of MS than their black neighbors. Even within the U.S., white people have two times the incidence of black people. The prevalence of MS in subpopulations of black Africans and their North American descendants correlates with their genetic intermixture with Caucasians. Hispanic Americans have rates of MS similar to black Americans. Native Americans have an even lower prevalence; like African Americans, their chance of being diagnosed with MS correlates with the extent of Caucasian ancestry. Because the incidence of MS is so low in these subpopulations, no recent rate data are available. Ongoing studies, however, are gathering incidence data for racial minorities in the U.S., and the information will be helpful both for explaining the rising incidence of MS in people of color and for comparing genetic details of various subgroups with MS.

Familial Distribution

The incidence of MS in people who have a blood relative with MS is higher than that in the general population. This confirms that there is a genetic component to the disease. For someone in the general population, the chance of getting MS is about one in a thousand. In comparison, the identical twin of a person with MS has a one in three chance of getting it, while nonidentical siblings of the affected person have a one in twenty to thirty chance. Studies of adopted siblings show that they have no increased risk, so the chance is low that increased risk within a family is due simply to a shared environment—there must be a genetic link. The lifetime risk for a sibling increases when the affected sibling is a brother, and if one or both parents have MS. The child of a person with MS has a one in forty chance of getting it. While these rates are much higher than for the general population, they are still

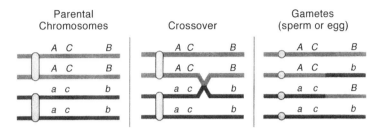

Figure 1.2 Crossing over between an individual's maternal and paternal chromosomes, which have just divided, during meiosis. Chromosomes are inherited in pairs. Genes that are close together on a chromosome, such as A and C, are more commonly inherited together than genes far apart, such as C and B, because recombination, or crossing over, is less likely to occur between them. This figure shows a crossover between genes C and B, where B and b are exchanged. Note that there are four possible gene combinations after recombination occurs, whereas there were only two combinations before

relatively low, and the fact that not all identical twins have MS means that factors other than genetics also play a role.

Two types of studies are commonly used to determine the contribution of heredity to MS: *linkage analysis* and *association studies*. Linkage analysis is based on the fact that genes close together on a chromosome tend to be inherited together, that is, they are physically linked. During meiosis, the biological process in which sperm and egg cells are produced, the arms of chromosomes cross over, exchanging DNA to mix the genes of the mother and father (see fig. 1.2). Because there is more chromosomal distance between genes that are far apart, crossovers occur more frequently between them. In contrast, genes that are close together are often exchanged together and inherited together. If a marker gene—one not directly involved in MS but easy to locate—consistently correlates with the occurrence of MS, then the genes linked to it are candidates for involvement in MS. Linkage analysis uses multiplex MS families (those in which several members have MS) to investigate correlations between MS and various genetic markers.

An association study determines whether or not a specific disease marker occurs more frequently in MS patients than in the general population. This type of analysis is essentially an expansion of a linkage analysis in which all members of the population are treated as distant relatives, inheriting their genes from a common ancestor. Association of a pair of genes requires that they be in linkage disequilibrium—that is, that they are inherited together more frequently than is expected by chance alone—and also is limited to the detection of disease genes very close to the marker gene. If a particular gene is found to be associated with the marker, it becomes a candidate for involvement in MS.

Both linkage analysis and association studies confirm the contribution of genetic factors to the incidence of MS.

Genetic Factors

Investigators are trying to determine which genes might confer susceptibility to MS. Each gene occurs at a unique location on a specific chromosome; once a "hot spot" is identified, the genes located at that spot can be analyzed for their correlation with the onset and progression of MS. Since MS is an autoimmune disease, many of the implicated genes are involved in triggering and propagating the immune response.

Genes are inherited in pairs, with different combinations being contributed by the father and the mother. Each gene within a pair is called an *allele*. Some alleles are dominant, which means that it only takes one copy for the encoded trait to be expressed. Examples of dominant genes are those that encode dark eye color and A or B blood type. Some alleles are recessive, meaning that two copies must be present for the encoded trait to be expressed. Examples of recessive traits are blue eyes and type O blood. Most genes have more than two unique alleles, due to a characteristic known as polymorphism. Polymorphism ("many forms") is the occurrence of different DNA sequences within the same gene. In humans, the group of genes with the highest amount of polymorphism also happens to be the group most closely associated with MS susceptibility.

Every gene encodes a specific trait, called a *phenotype*. Some phenotypes, such as skin color and height, are obvious to the naked eye. Other phenotypes, such as which receptors are on your taste buds and how efficient your metabolism is, are only detectable at the molecular level. The phenotypes of MS-associated genes are of the latter sort, and only analyses of the genes themselves or the proteins they encode can shed light on the relationship between heredity and clinical disease.

Many phenotypes are interrelated, and some can mask others. The masking effect is called *epistasis*, an example of which is the Bombay phenotype. In this condition, people who possess genes for A or B blood type actually express the O blood type, due to a mutation that causes the A or B precursor protein to be incompletely formed. In an epistasis group, several genes produce proteins that can mask the mutation or loss of one of the other proteins from the group. This is why all possible manifestations of a gene might not be observed. The term describing this is *penetrance*. Penetrance is the proportion of individuals who have a particular gene that actually expresses the trait associated with that gene. Penetrance is low for all the MS-associated genes studied so far. This means that, while all MS patients may have a particular gene, all people with that gene do not necessarily have MS. Researchers are still looking for additional genes whose penetrance is high and for combinations of genes that result in higher penetrance than any individual gene alone.

The only genes definitely associated with MS susceptibility are collectively known as the *human leukocyte antigen (HLA) complex*. HLA proteins play a role in inducing inflammation by activating T cells to attack and destroy diseased cells nearby (see chapter 2). The inflammatory immune response rids the body of foreign substances such as bacteria and viruses, but it can also harm tissues. In the case of autoimmune diseases, a person's own tissues are both the trigger and the target of the attack, causing a variety of symptoms ranging from pain (associated with MS) to high blood sugar (associated with Type 1 diabetes).

The location, or *locus*, of the HLA complex is on the short arm of chromosome 6. It comprises more than four million base pairs (the whole chromosome comprises 183 million base pairs) and represents more than 200 different genes. HLA genes code for proteins in two main classes, I and II, which present peptides of different lengths to T cells. The classes are further divided into subtypes: A, B, C, E, F, and G for class I, and subtype D for class II. Forty percent of the genes at this locus are involved in the immune system, and most are polymorphic, like HLA-B of class I, which has almost 450 known alleles.

HLA proteins are considered antigens because they can produce an immune response in an organ recipient. Incompatibility of HLA alleles is the reason for transplant rejection. Similarly, the HLA proteins in the host can be recognized as foreign by immune cells in the transplant and cause graft-versus-host disease. The process of matching transplant donor and potential recipient involves making sure their HLA alleles are compatible. It is possible that HLA proteins play an analogous role in inducing autoimmunity, where a person's own tissues are recognized and attacked as if they were foreign.

Several other genes have been investigated for their association with MS, including (1) genes for the T cell receptor, the molecule on the T cell surface that interacts with HLA proteins, (2) genes encoding immunoglobulins, better known as antibodies, which are analogous to the T cell receptor except that they are found both in soluble form and on the surface of particular immune cells, and (3) genes encoding myelin structural proteins, which make up the protective sheath surrounding the nerves. None of these genes has been associated directly with MS susceptibility, but each of them is certainly involved in the progression of MS. Studying these genes in more detail will help shed light on the mechanisms of MS progression so that, one day, investigators may be able to correlate a genetic pattern with the course of the disease.

Environmental Factors

For several decades it has been observed that the incidence of MS increases with increasing distance from the equator (see fig. 1.3). This points to an environmental factor as being important in triggering the onset of the disease. While the north-south gradient of incidence is not as pronounced as it has been in the past, the immigration effect is well established, and further supports an environmental cause for MS.

The immigration effect is seen when a population group living in a region of low MS incidence relocates to a place where MS incidence is high. Studies show that if the relocation happens before puberty, the immigrant population acquires the MS risk of the new home. The same is true for those who move from high-risk to low-risk areas. Investigators who favor an environmental cause for MS hypothesize that an unknown trigger, perhaps a virus, infects people during a

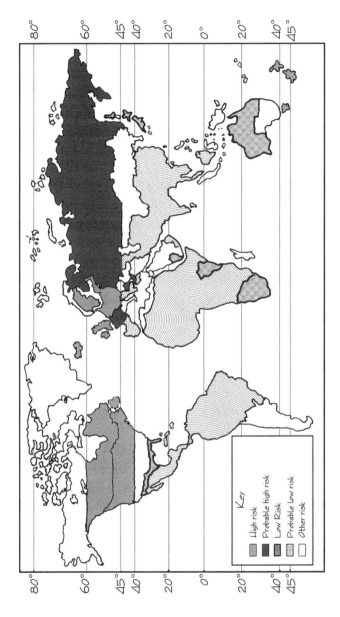

Figure 1.3 Map showing the worldwide occurrence of MS

window of opportunity in prepubescence, and that it has an incubation period of years before it becomes manifest.

One way to discover specific environmental contributors is to study *clusters*, small segments of the population that have an unusually high incidence of MS. The first cluster to be recorded was in the Faroe Islands, located between Norway and Iceland in the northern Atlantic Ocean. The British occupied the area during World War II. Prior to that, MS was unknown there (at least, it was never diagnosed). During 1943, rates of MS among the natives jumped to ten in 100,000. The increased incidence corresponded almost exactly with the occupied towns. Three additional distinct surges in MS rates have occurred since then, in 1955, 1969, and 1986. One interpretation of these MS epidemics is that the British soldiers harbored an infectious agent that, when released in the Faroes, went through a dormant period before emerging some years later as MS. The cyclic nature of the increases in incidence suggests that the incubation period is about fourteen years.

Epidemics of MS like those observed in the Faroe Islands lend support to the theory that an environmental substance may trigger the disease. The most likely candidate is a virus. Several viruses have been investigated for their effect on MS, including measles, herpes, influenza, and even rabies. Researchers have failed to demonstrate that any of these has a direct causal relationship with MS, though in some studies viral particles were found to be coincident with MS symptoms.

The causes of MS cannot be entirely environmental, because different racial groups living together do not have the same rates of incidence. Nor can they be entirely genetic, because concordance in identical twins is only partial, and investigators have yet to determine a full array of genes that render a person susceptible to MS. The fact that MS prevalence increases with latitude indicates an environmental component, and the high incidence within certain families indicates a genetic component. Thus, there is not one specific gene that causes MS, but several acting together that increase susceptibility, and an environmental factor triggers the disease process.

2. What is MS?

MS is a disease in which the immune system damages the insulation around nerve cells. Loss of this insulation causes nerve impulses to slow down and eventually stop. Because the effects of MS do not become evident until substantial damage has occurred, people in the early stages of MS often look completely healthy. What is happening in the body during this "silent" period? When do the effects of the damage become apparent? This chapter will describe the normal functions of the central nervous system and the immune system and explain how they interact in an aberrant manner to cause the disease we call multiple sclerosis.

The Central Nervous System

The *central nervous system (CNS)* comprises the brain and the spinal cord. These organs are responsible for coordinating the senses of touch, taste, smell, sight, and hearing with appropriate responses. The CNS is composed of two main cell types: *neurons* and the cells that support them, called *glia*. There are three types of glial cells in the CNS—astrocytes, oligodendrocytes, and microglia—constituting about 50 percent of the total cell count.

Different types of neurons conduct signals to, from, and within the CNS. Sensory neurons transmit signals from the five sense organs to the CNS. Motor neurons send signals from the CNS to a muscle or a gland, telling it what to do. Association neurons link the signals between sensory and motor neurons within the CNS.

Structurally, neurons possess dendrites, which project out from the cell body to sense incoming nerve signals, and axons, which transmit those signals to other neurons or to effector organs (see fig. 2.1). Just as electrical wires are insulated for efficient energy conduction, so are neurons. The insulating material is called *myelin* and is produced by the oligodendrocytes. Myelin is composed of specialized lipids and proteins that allow it to adhere to itself and to the axon with which it is associated. The gaps between myelinated segments of an axon are called nodes of Ranvier. At the nodes, the axon wall contains protein channels where ions flow into and out of the axon.

Neurons can be stimulated by mechanical force, pain, heat, light, or chemicals. Stimulation beyond a certain threshold creates an electrical cascade, called an *action potential*, within the associated axon, causing ion channels in the axonal membrane to open and allow sodium ions to flow into the neuron and potassium ions to flow out. The resulting local alteration in charge distribution is, in turn, a stimulus for the opening of ion channels at the next node of Ranvier. Ions move along the myelinated segment of the axon to the next node to trigger the action potential there. Once an ion channel is opened, it is refractory, or incapable of responding to further stimuli, for a brief period of time. The refractory period allows propagation of the action potential in one direction, away from the dendrites and toward the terminal end of the axon. Myelination increases the speed of action potential propagation by allowing the electrical impulse to "jump" from node to node.

The CNS is insulated from the rest of the body by tightly spaced endothelial cells that line the capillaries in the brain. This lining, called the *blood-brain barrier (BBB)*, selects the types of molecules and cells that can pass into brain tissue. The BBB is reinforced by astrocytes, the most abundant glial

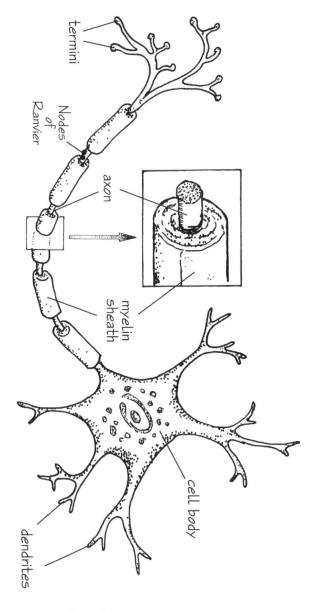

Figure 2.1 A myelinated neuron

cell type. Astrocyte extensions called perivascular feet almost completely surround the capillaries. The close association of astrocytes with the BBB positions them for a strategic role: the recruitment of immune cells into the CNS.

The Immune System

The body is able to recognize itself. It distinguishes its own cells from other cells by the unique molecular markers displayed on their surfaces. The body can tell when foreign cells are present, as in an organ transplant, or when a pathogen (a virus, bacterium, fungus, or parasite) has entered it. The immune system is the network of organs, tissues, cells, and biomolecules that defends the body against things that are "nonself." The immune system recognizes a foreign substance and mounts a cellular and molecular response to rid the body of it.

Immunity is divided into two classes: innate and acquired. *Innate immunity* is the body's first line of defense. It responds to a wide variety of foreign substances and has nonspecific recognition mechanisms. *Acquired immunity*, also called *adaptive immunity*, is specific for a particular foreign agent and is characterized by the ability to "remember" that agent so that the second and subsequent responses to it are increasingly effective. Both types of immunity require the concerted action of many cell types and signaling molecules.

Most immune cells fall into the category of leukocytes, or white blood cells. These are further subdivided into phagocytes, lymphocytes, and auxiliary cells. Each cell type has unique mechanisms for detecting and interacting with antigens, the immune-stimulating components of foreign substances. Each immune cell is also able to interact with other immune cells to heighten or suppress the immune response.

Phagocytes ("eating cells") mediate the innate immune response. They rid the body of invaders by ingesting them. *Macrophages* and *dendritic cells* are "professional" phagocytes whose specific surface receptors allow them to recognize various antigens. Phagocytes in the brain are called *microglia*. Phagocytic cells have the ability to break down ingested foreign agents into their molecular components and display them as antigens for recognition by T cells. In this capacity, they are called *antigen-presenting cells (APCs)*.

The acquired immune response depends on lymphocytes, primarily B cells and T cells. B cells, which originate in the bone marrow, display immunoglobulin proteins, or antibodies, on their surfaces. When those antibodies recognize antigens, it activates B cells to secrete soluble forms of the antibodies. Soluble antibodies facilitate the immune response by binding to and immobilizing antigens, targeting them for degradation by phagocytes.

T cells, which also originate in bone marrow, but mature in the thymus, have a wider range of activities. Some T cells interact with phagocytes to help them destroy pathogens. Others recognize virally infected cells and kill them directly. Still others are involved in controlling antibody production by B cells.

Antigen Recognition and Presentation

All immune cells have the ability to recognize antigens. B cells interact with antigens through the antibodies displayed on their surfaces. Antibodies are proteins composed of four separate amino acid chains—two light and two heavy. The heavy and light chains are held together by covalent bonds, disulfide bonds, between pairs of sulfur atoms. The structural organization of the amino acid chains gives antibodies a

Y shape. Individual chains are genetically encoded to have variable amino acid sequences at locations corresponding to the tips of the Y, where the antibody interacts with antigens. Each B cell makes antibody with a single sequence, and that antibody recognizes a single antigen. There are enough B cells in the immune system to recognize and respond to millions of different antigens.

T cells recognize antigens via their characteristic cell surface protein—the T cell receptor (TCR). The TCR is organized with two amino acid chains held together by a disulfide bond, plus several accessory proteins that are essential for its function. Like an antibody, the TCR has variable amino acid sequences at its tip. However, whereas antibodies recognize antigens in their full molecular form, the TCR can only recognize antigen fragments, and only in the context of a human leukocyte antigen (HLA) molecule from another immune cell. This is the process performed by antigen-presenting phagocytes.

During antigen presentation, APCs break down antigenic molecules into small fragments, called *epitopes*. The epitopes are packaged within a groove on the tip of the HLA molecules displayed by APCs. The TCR binds to the HLA and is introduced to the epitope it contains. The T cell whose TCR meets the epitope is triggered to stimulate an immune response against antigens containing that epitope.

Antigen recognition by lymphocytes triggers several events. Phagocytes are activated to ingest the entire foreign body on which the antigen is displayed. For instance, if a bacterial cell displays one antigenic protein molecule, the whole cell will be engulfed and digested. B cells are stimulated to release soluble antibodies, which seek out soluble antigens and mark them for degradation by phagocytes. T cells begin releasing signaling molecules called *cytokines*, which affect the metabolism, localization, and function of both the T cell itself and surrounding cells.

Cytokines are the messengers of the immune system. Specific combinations of cytokines direct various leukocytes to proliferate, differentiate, migrate, or produce more or different cytokines. Cytokines can be classified into several families of proteins. The *interferons* are the first line of defense against viral infections, inducing a state of viral resistance in uninfected cells. *Interleukins* are the largest cytokine family. Most interleukins are involved in cell division and differentiation, and each one is specific for a particular type of immune cell. *Colony stimulating factors* promote differentiation of white blood cells both within and outside the bone marrow. Various interleukins, as well as interferon-gamma and a cytokine called tumor necrosis factor, are involved in the inflammatory response.

Inflammation

Several auxiliary cell types mediate inflammation, the process by which leukocytes are attracted to a site of infection. Inflammation is characterized by an increase in blood supply, bringing leukocytes to the infected area, and vascular permeability, allowing leukocytes and signaling molecules to pass into and out of the infected tissue. Inflammation is triggered by recognition of an antigen, which results in the migration of phagocytes to the site of infection. Phagocytes then release cytokines, whose job is to initiate inflammation by stimulating the proliferation and differentiation of lymphocytes and phagocytes and recruiting them to the infected tissue. Once the infection is successfully eradicated, inflammation is stopped by the programmed death of transient populations of immune cells. The system returns to its resting state and performs routine surveillance in anticipation of the next invasion.

Immune surveillance takes place via the interface between the circulatory system and the lymphatic system (see fig. 2.2). Immune cells originate and develop in the lymphatic organs, primarily the thymus and the bone marrow. From there, they migrate to the secondary lymphoid organs: the spleen, the lymph nodes, and the mucosal tissues. The lymphoid organs and tissues are connected by a network of vessels through which immune cells circulate. The lymphatic vessels interface with the circulatory system in the lymph nodes, where immune cells pass into and out of the bloodstream. Foreign agents entering the body through the skin, the lungs, or the intestines are recognized in the mucosal tissues. Activated lymphocytes migrate from there to the lymph nodes to recruit other immune cells to fight the invader.

The recruitment of lymphocytes and phagocytes to the site of an infection is mediated by adhesion proteins expressed on the surface of both immune cells and the endothelial cells that line the vasculature. *Cellular adhesion molecules (CAMs)* are displayed exclusively on vascular endothelial cells. *Integrins* and *selectins* are found on both leukocytes and endothelial cells. The chemical properties of these proteins, including electronic charge and overall shape, allow them to stick to each other. Carbohydrate molecules are also involved as binding partners for some of these adhesion proteins.

Immune cells migrate into an infected tissue in a multistep process that utilizes each class of adhesion molecule (see fig. 2.3). Intercellular adhesion is initiated by tethering, where circulating leukocytes are slowed down by the interactions between selectins and carbohydrates on leukocytes and epithelial cells, respectively. Tethering is followed by triggering, in

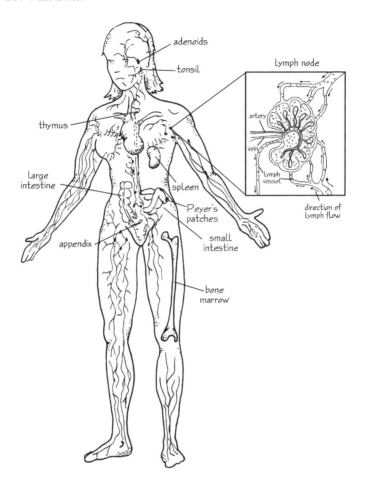

Figure 2.2 The lymphatic system and its interface with the circulatory system in the lymph nodes. The primary and secondary lymphatic organs are labeled, and the general structure of a lymph node is shown in the expansion. The fluid flowing through the lymphatic system is called lymph

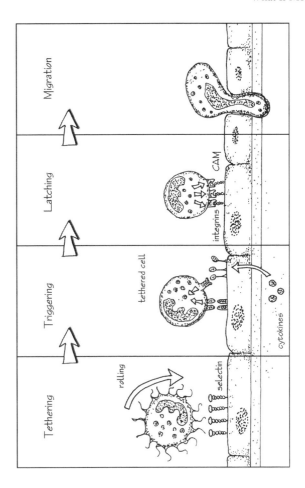

Figure 2.3 Steps of cell adhesion. Selectins mediate tethering, cytokines mediate triggering, and integrins and CAMs mediate latching. Migration occurs when the circulating cell squeezes between epithelial cells and moves into the surrounding tissue

which arrested leukocytes are stimulated to migrate across the epithelium by expression of cytokines from the cell to which they have adhered. Latching and activation involve the production of high-affinity integrins on the leukocytes, which bind to the CAMs on the epithelium and begin the migration process. Migration across the epithelium into the tissue then proceeds as the immune cells roll along the surface of the epithelial cells using additional adhesion proteins.

Immunity in the CNS

Since the CNS is sequestered away from the rest of the body by the BBB, how does the immune system fight infections when they occur within the CNS? How do leukocytes get past the BBB? Specialized immune cells reside within the CNS and trigger an immune response that permeabilizes the BBB.

Astrocytes are the most abundant type of glial cell in the CNS. As described previously, they surround the endothelial cells that compose the BBB. Astrocytes permeabilize the BBB by secreting a cytokine called tumor necrosis factor-alpha. Tumor necrosis factor-alpha stimulates astrocytes to express intercellular adhesion molecules, which aid the migration of circulating leukocytes into the brain. Astrocytes also secrete cytokines that attract T cells to the site of inflammation.

A second type of immune cell in the CNS is the microglial cell. Microglia constitute up to 20 percent of the cells in the CNS and can respond to antigens like circulating phagocytes. In response to cytokines, microglia proliferate and migrate to the site of an infection. Activation of microglial cells stimulates their production of human leukocyte antigen, which prepares them to become APCs.

Autoimmunity and MS

It is critical for the immune system to distinguish between self-derived (autologous) molecules and foreign (exogenous) molecules. Autoimmunity is the state in which the immune system confuses self and foreign molecules and launches an attack against self molecules. The systems that regulate self-recognition break down, and phagocytes begin to ingest a person's own healthy cells. Examples of common autoimmune diseases include type I diabetes and rheumatoid arthritis.

Acceptance of self molecules is called tolerance and is programmed into developing populations of T cells and B cells. Self-reactive lymphocytes are usually killed off during their maturation in the lymphatic system, but a small number survive and are present in the adult. These self-reactive cells can be activated by the presentation of self antigens.

The prevailing theory of autoimmunity in MS is that myelin component proteins act as autologous antigens. APCs present myelin epitopes to T cells, which stimulates the production of anti-myelin antibodies by B cells. The inflammatory response brings phagocytes to the site of antigen recognition—the brain, in the case of MS—and the oligodendrocytes that produce myelin are attacked and killed.

What causes APCs to present myelin epitopes as if they were foreign? Three hypotheses address this question:

- *Epitope spreading.* This hypothesis states that a chronic viral infection induces a normal immune response in which phagocytes break down infected tissues. The damaged tissue releases autologous molecules that are recognized by the rare self-reactive T cell. The self-recognition triggers a secondary immune response against the source of the self antigen.

• *Molecular mimicry*. This hypothesis holds that certain viral epitopes are structurally similar to host epitopes. The similarity is great enough that T cells recognizing the viral epitope are also activated against the host epitope.
• *Bystander activation*. This hypothesis explains the activation of self-reactive T cells as the result of cytokine release during the inflammatory response against an invader. Self-reactive T cells are activated along with the rest of the local T cell population and, if they happen to recognize a self antigen, an autoimmune response is generated. Bystander activation explains how some autoimmune diseases seem to be triggered by viral infection when there is no evidence of cross-reactivity between viral and autologous epitopes.

Multiple sclerosis means "many scars," because inflammatory episodes leave behind visible damage in the CNS. The scars, called *plaques*, are visible as discolorations in the myelinated white matter of the brain. At the cellular level, the effect of myelin breakdown is to slow down nerve impulses. As a result, people with MS experience one or more symptoms, including pain, numbness, tingling, or visual disturbances. The recurring cycle of inflammatory demyelination leads eventually to neuronal degeneration and loss of mobility.

3. Symptoms and Diagnosis of MS

"But you look so good!" This is a reaction MS patients commonly receive from family members, friends, and even physicians. The invisible signs and symptoms of MS may make it hard for some people to believe there is a real illness occurring. Symptoms like slight numbness or fatigue may be confused with everyday experiences. Further complications arise when clinical observations of MS plaques do not correlate with the appearance or progression of symptoms. Fortunately for MS patients today, criteria are in place to help them describe and categorize their symptoms and their particular type of MS. While diagnosis of this disease is still longer in coming than for most other illnesses, a combination of both laboratory and clinical tests can usually confirm that MS is or is not occurring.

History of MS Diagnosis

The earliest descriptions of MS date back to the Middle Ages. Journal entries preserved from the eighteenth and nineteenth centuries detail discrete episodes of pain, loss of vision or balance, and incontinence. Doctors in those times relied solely upon observation of the patient to diagnose a disease, and only after death, if an autopsy was performed, were the underlying causes of symptoms discovered. Still, MS was distinct enough in its manifestations to be comprehensively described by Jean-Martin Charcot in a series of lectures at the University of Paris in 1872–1873. Charcot is known as "the father of neurology" and produced many drawings from autopsies he performed. These illustrations gave the first real description of the physical changes that accompany MS.

The invention of the electron microscope early in the twentieth century gave scientists a closer look at cells in the nervous system, and they began to define the activity of nerve cells using newly developed electrophysical techniques. Also, the advent of vaccination against viral diseases, particularly rabies, produced a small number of adverse reactions characterized by MS-like symptoms, leading to the still prevalent theory that there is a viral trigger for MS. The connection between immunity and the central nervous system was firmly established in 1947 by Dr. Elvin Kabat during the first research study funded by the National MS Society. Most recently, advances in imaging technology, primarily magnetic resonance imaging (MRI), have helped doctors diagnose the disease earlier and with more certainty. Images of the brain have given investigators insight into the underlying progression of MS, providing the basic knowledge needed to effectively combat the disease.

Early Symptoms

Symptoms of MS are categorized as primary, secondary, and tertiary. Primary symptoms are those caused directly by the demyelination process. All the symptoms described in this chapter are primary symptoms, including vision problems, fatigue, and weakness. Secondary symptoms are ailments caused by the effects of MS. For example, primary bladder problems can cause persistent urinary tract infections, or the loss of movement in an arm or leg can result in muscle deterioration.

Tertiary symptoms are the social, emotional, and vocational effects of primary and secondary symptoms. MS causes stress for all involved, from the patient and the family to their friends and co-workers. Coping with the relational challenges arising from having MS is discussed in chapter 5.

In this section, I describe symptoms that usually occur early on in the progression of MS. These are often problems that are addressed in the first series of visits to the doctor before the patient knows what is wrong and before a diagnosis has been made. Early symptoms often persist into later stages of the disease and may eventually become peripheral to or masked by other more uncomfortable symptoms that occur as demyelination progresses.

Numbness

Numbness involves a localized loss of sensation or a tingling feeling. It is one of the first symptoms experienced by MS patients and is sometimes described as feeling "pins and needles." Numbness may be mild or may be severe enough to affect the use of the numbed body part. This symptom requires extra caution on the part of the MS patient to avoid injury from heat, utensils, or oneself.

Weakness and Spasticity

Weakness, usually described as limited muscle capacity, affects about 80 percent of MS patients. Legs are affected more often than arms, usually not to an equal extent. Some people report weakness in only one leg or in a leg and an arm on the same side of the body. Weakness often occurs in conjunction with other MS symptoms, such as tremor, ataxia (loss of coordination), and, most commonly, spasticity. *Spasticity* is a state of muscular contraction in which the muscle resists passive movement (movement induced by an external force). Muscle spasms in MS are sometimes strong enough to cause pain, and they can even eject a person from a wheelchair. The mechanisms and effects of weakness and spasticity in MS are similar to those in spinal-cord injuries. Both physical injury and demyelination cause a decrease in the rate and strength of nerve conduction through the spinal cord. Individual nerves conduct impulses more slowly, and the complete loss of some axons means that fewer nerves are stimulating a single muscle. Muscle contraction requires reaching a threshold nerve potential, and there may simply not be enough active nerves to reach this threshold. Eventually, the lack of muscle innervation and muscular contraction produces muscle deterioration and shortening of the muscle fibers. In some cases, joint deformities result.

Vision Problems

Visual disturbances of some kind occur in a majority of people with MS. These symptoms are the very first manifestation in about 35 percent of patients. They can include inflammation of the optic nerve (optic neuritis), blurred vision, and abnormal eye movements. With *optic neuritis*, a person may experience vision loss, painful eye movements, dimmed vision, or altered depth perception. The symptoms usually persist up to one week, followed by a period of recovery over several weeks or months. It is estimated that a person with optic neuritis has a 45 to 80 percent chance of being diagnosed with MS within fifteen years.

Poor Coordination

Ataxia, a lack of coordination, always occurs in conjunction with tremor, an involuntary, rhythmic movement, usually of one arm. Ataxia can also affect the legs, in which case the person's ability to stand or walk is compromised. Sensory ataxia occurs when a person cannot feel their feet well enough to place them correctly. Weakness in the leg muscles is also a common cause of gait problems. As with muscular weakness, loss of coordination can be seen in either one leg (monoparesis) or both legs (paraparesis). At first the main consequence of these symptoms is embarrassment, but as the symptoms worsen, the person with MS may be at risk for an injury if there is no support from another person or an assistive device.

Diagnosis

Because symptoms and clinical manifestations vary widely between people with MS, diagnosis has been a trouble spot in treating people. Diagnostic criteria have been developed slowly over the last few decades, with each new set of criteria incorporating the scientific understanding and technological advances available at the time. In 2001, a new consensus was reached regarding what symptoms should be present and what clinical tests should be done to reach a positive diagnosis.

Demographic Profile

The physician records a detailed history of the patient's health, including a description of current symptoms and any past or present attacks experienced. The demographic profile of the patient is considered, since MS occurs in demographic tiers as discussed in chapter 1. Age, sex, race, family history, and geographic location are all factors that may help confirm the indications of clinical testing. They may be useful for differentiating MS from other neurological diseases, such as amyotrophic lateral sclerosis (ALS, Lou Gehrig's disease) and muscular dystrophy, that exhibit similar symptoms.

Laboratory Profile

A laboratory profile of the patient includes magnetic resonance imaging (MRI). MRI exams are used to create cross-sectional images of the brain. Lesions in brain tissue can be detected with a variety of MRI methods. Gadolinium is sometimes administered to increase the visual contrast between tissues. Since this element is normally excluded from the brain, its entry into brain tissue is indicative of inflammation-induced breakdown of the blood-brain barrier. Another compound, N-acetyl aspartate, a simple derivative of a common amino acid, is found only in brain axons and neurons. Reduced levels of N-acetyl aspartate can be detected by magnetic resonance spectra and correlate in general with loss of neural activity (and with specific symptoms for some types of MS). Other MRI methods measure the cumulative burden of disease or give an overall indication of the extent of tissue damage. The combination of multiple methods is crucial to obtaining a positive diagnosis.

Standard laboratory testing also includes analysis of the cerebrospinal fluid (CSF) for increased antibody production. The result most commonly associated with MS is the detection of oligoclonal bands, so called because of their appearance in a polyacrylamide gel matrix to which an electric charge has been applied. The term *oligoclonal* (oligo = a few; clone = cells derived from a single parent cell) refers to the fact that several bands are present, each corresponding to a different immuno-globulin protein. The presence in CSF of immunoglobulin protein bands that are absent from the blood is considered a positive sign of immune activity in the CNS. Diseases other than MS can also produce these bands, so the presence of oligo-clonal bands is typical of but not exclusive to MS CSF.

Clinical Profile

Finally, the clinical profile is assessed. This includes the record and description of the number of attacks, the symptoms, and measurement of the neurological responsiveness of the patient.

An MS attack, also called an *exacerbation*, is a brief period of time in which MS symptoms are unmistakably worse. In the initial stages of the disease, attacks are obvious because patients are comparing the first MS symptoms with their normal physi-cal state. Loss of function in the arms or legs is common, as is extreme muscle weakness. After an increase in disability over time, the types of symptoms experienced during a relapse may change because sensory skills are less acute. To be considered a true attack, the symptoms must persist for at least twenty-four hours and be followed by a recovery period, usually lasting days or weeks. Separate attacks are defined as those having at least one month of stable physical activity between them.

Criteria

Established criteria for a positive diagnosis of MS include the number of attacks in combination with the amount of clinical and laboratory evidence. Until 2001, the most commonly used criteria were those introduced in 1983 by C. M. Poser and colleagues. The more recent McDonald criteria (see table 3.1) take into account the results from magnetic resonance imaging.

Classification

As MS progression in a patient becomes more and more evident, it can be classified according to several existing models and treated accordingly. The four major types of MS are *relapsing-remitting*, *secondary progressive*, *progressive relapsing*, and *primary progressive*. Figure 3.1 illustrates the chronological progression of MS in each subtype of the disease.

Relapsing-remitting MS (see fig. 3.1A) is characterized by distinct periods of acute inflammation that cause temporary flare-ups of symptoms, separated by periods of full recovery. About 85 percent of MS patients start out with this type, and 55 percent of people with MS retain this pattern of disease activity. This type is most responsive to disease-modifying therapies (see chapter 4).

Secondary progressive MS (see fig. 3.1B) begins the same way as relapsing-remitting MS, with intermittent attacks and periods of full recovery. Over time, however, the patient begins to retain disability after each attack. Many MS patients progress from relapsing MS to progressive MS, making this the second most common type of the disease (about 30 percent of people with MS are in this category). Paradoxically, these patients usually show less inflammatory activity than those with relapsing MS.

Progressive relapsing MS (see fig. 3.1C) is rare, accounting for about 5 percent of MS patients. This class is characterized by slow worsening and increasing disability from the onset of

Table 3.1 Diagnostic Criteria for Multiple Sclerosis[a]

Clinical Presentation	Additional Data Needed
• 2 or more attacks[b] • 2 or more objective clinical lesions	None; clinical evidence will suffice (additional evidence desirable but must be consistent with MS)
• 2 or more attacks • 1 objective clinical lesion	Dissemination in *space*, demonstrated by • MRI, **or** • a positive CSF[c] and 2 or more MRI lesions consistent with MS, **or** • further clinical attack involving different site
• 1 attack • 2 or more objective clinical lesions	Dissemination in *time*, demonstrated by • MRI, **or** • second clinical attack
• 1 attack • 1 objective clinical lesion	Dissemination in *space*, demonstrated by • MRI, **or** • a positive CSF and 2 or more MRI lesions consistent with MS **AND** Dissemination in *time*, demonstrated by • MRI, **or** • second clinical attack
• Insidious neurological progression suggestive of MS	Positive CSF **AND** Dissemination in *space*, demonstrated by • MRI evidence of 9 or more brain lesions, **or** • 2 or more spinal cord lesions, **or** • 4–8 brain and 1 spinal cord lesion, **or** • positive VEP[d] with 4–8 MRI lesions, **or** • positive VEP with <4 brain lesions plus 1 spinal cord lesion **AND** Dissemination in *time*, demonstrated by • MRI, **or** • continued progression for 1 year

[a]McDonald et al. Recommended diagnostic criteria for multiple sclerosis: guidelines from the International Panel on the diagnosis of multiple sclerosis. *Ann. Neurol.* 2001 Jul:50(1):121–7.
[b]An attack is defined as a reported or observed neurological disturbance of 24 hours minimum duration.
[c]CSF = cerebrospinal fluid. A positive CSF means the detection of immunoglobulins, i.e., oligoclonal bands.
[d]VEP = visually evoked potential. A test for slow conduction along the optic nerve.

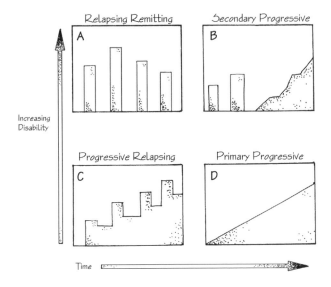

Figure 3.1 Time course of disease activity for different subtypes of MS. (A) Relapsing-remitting, (B) secondary progressive, (C) progressive relapsing, and (D) primary progressive subtypes are depicted

the disease. Acute attacks of increasing severity are superimposed on the progression of this type of MS.

Primary progressive MS (see fig. 3.1D) is also characterized by slow worsening of symptoms, but without the acute attacks. About 10 percent of MS patients are in this category. This MS subtype is more often found in patients who are older than average at onset, and the male:female ratio is greatest for this type of MS.

Later Symptoms

As MS progresses, new symptoms become more noticeable. Initial symptoms are linked directly to inflammatory activity in the CNS, whereas later symptoms develop as the result of lost axonal activity.

Pain

As MS progresses and as the patient ages, pain is likely to become a symptom. Women are more prone to experience pain than men. Manifestations of pain come in a wide variety, some being associated with acute MS attacks and others persisting continuously. Many physicians believe that if the disease process can be stopped, so can the pain, but currently available treatments have limited effect on this troubling symptom.

Pain is categorized as *neuropathic, acute due to inflammation, secondary to increased muscle tone*, or *chronic nonspecific*. Neuropathic pain syndromes, those due to neurodegeneration, include trigeminal neuralgia—a brief shock-like sensation, commonly experienced by the elderly, which can be triggered by specific localized touch at certain points on the face—and tonic spasms, which are severe muscle contractions triggered by movement or general sensory stimulation. Tonic spasms occur very rarely in the general population and thus are highly correlated to the activity of MS. The most common neuropathic pain in MS is a burning sensation called dysesthetic pain. It is usually felt in the lower extremities, and sensory defects overlap with the location of the pain.

Pain due directly to MS-related inflammation is exemplified by optic neuritis. This aching pain accompanies the visual disturbances characteristic of optic neuritis and is exacerbated by eye movements. Pain that occurs secondary to increased muscle tone is directly related to spasticity and usually improves if the spasticity is treated. Chronic nonspecific pain includes neck or back pain and may be caused by other MS symptoms, such as muscle weakness or abnormal gait. This type of pain is commonly experienced in the general population, making it difficult to correlate with MS itself. The same is true for headache, although enough studies have been done to establish a relationship between MS and this common malady. Headache occurs in 52 percent of MS patients, a much higher incidence than is found in the general population. Headache does not necessarily correlate with clinical exacerbations, but in a few patients it does precede the onset of an attack.

Cognitive Dysfunction

Cognitive dysfunction refers to a decreased ability to think, reason, concentrate, or remember. The symptom is seen in about half of MS patients, sometimes early enough to be included as a first symptom. Only a small percentage of people with MS have cognitive problems severe enough to cause significant changes in their daily lives. The level of cognitive dysfunction correlates with the degree of demyelination in the brain, which supports the view that MS can directly cause slowing of thought processes. However, MS can also affect cognition indirectly, following from the mental stress, anxiety, depression, or other mental conditions experienced as a result of being diagnosed with MS. These symptoms can also affect the ability to think clearly and remember accurately. Like other MS symptoms, cognitive disorders vary between people. The most common disruption is a decline in memory, especially the ability to find the right words. This may or may not occur to a noticeable extent, since most people struggle to find the right word from time to time.

Fatigue

Fatigue is defined as an overwhelming sense of tiredness or exhaustion or a general lack of energy. It is felt as a result of, or in anticipation of, both physical and mental tasks, such as an exercise routine or a social engagement that requires concentration. Fatigue is often hard to differentiate from related MS symptoms such as true muscle weakness or depression.

In research studies, fatigue has not been linked directly to the biological activity of MS, but correlates more to psychological factors such as stress and mental effort. Its effects are worsened by heat, perhaps because movement of weak limbs is more difficult at higher temperatures. Fatigue is experienced by up to 90 percent of MS patients, most of whom report having to battle it on a daily basis. It is impartial to the age of the MS patient and the level of disability.

Fatigue is measured clinically in four components: behavior, perception, physiological mechanism, and context. Behavioral measurements refer to the loss of ability to complete a routine task, either physical or mental. Perception of fatigue is, of course, how difficult the patient perceives a certain task to be. Perception of fatigue can occur even when the task does not actually have to be done. Mechanisms of fatigue are usually measured from observations of peripheral nerve or muscle activity. Contextual measurements rate the influence of environment, including temperature, noise levels, and people, on the perception and mechanisms of fatigue.

Bladder and Bowel Problems

Bladder dysfunction is the first symptom in only 5 percent of MS patients, but its prevalence correlates with progression of the disease, eventually affecting up to 90 percent of all MS patients. Bowel dysfunction affects as many as 68 percent of people with MS, and it may be related to bladder dysfunction in that people with the latter are hesitant to drink sufficient fluids, leading to constipation. Signs of bladder dysfunction include a frequent and/or urgent need to urinate, involuntary urination, difficulty initiating or completing urination, a sense of urine retention, and incontinence during sleep. The mechanisms causing bladder dysfunction involve an interconnected system of nerves and muscles that coordinate the contraction and relaxation of the muscles that allow for normal urination. Many treatments are available that target specific aspects of these mechanisms and make symptoms manageable, although progression of the disease may result in the eventual need for catheterization.

Less is known about the mechanisms causing bowel dysfunction. Its symptoms include constipation and fecal incontinence, which affect about 50 percent and 30 percent of MS patients, respectively. Treatments are few and usually have undesirable side effects. More research is needed on the basic neurobiology of the gastrointestinal tract before new therapies can be designed.

4. MS Treatments

People with MS have more treatment options today than ever before. Disease progression can be delayed with one of several disease-modifying drugs. These compounds, along with corticosteroids, can effectively stop exacerbations caused by CNS inflammation and reduce their occurrence. This chapter will review the drug treatments available for MS and its symptoms. The final section addresses alternative methods of treating MS.

History of MS Treatment

It could be said that the history of MS parallels the history of medicine as a whole. Every breakthrough in thought, practice, or technology has been applied to diagnosing or treating the disease. Whereas the life expectancy of an MS patient in 1900 was just five years, it is now ten times that, provided the symptoms are recognized early and treatment is begun.

Throughout the 1950s, new discoveries in basic science led to a more thorough understanding of the organization and function of the central nervous system. But there were more questions than answers, due to the lack of scientifically controlled studies on the effectiveness of new therapies. At that time, MS was still most often treated by anticoagulants (blood "thinners"), because it was thought to be caused by circulation abnormalities. The first controlled clinical trial was conducted in the 1960s with adrenocorticotropic hormone (ACTH), a natural steroid that suppresses inflammation. Individuals treated with ACTH recovered from an MS attack faster than those who received a placebo.

ACTH was the first of several drugs discovered to slow the progress of MS. As early as the 1970s, beta-interferon and copolymer-1 were tested for their effectiveness in delaying the progression of MS; they are still marketed today under the names of Betaseron and Copaxone. The so-called disease-modifying drugs can now be combined with more specialized ones that target the symptoms, such as fatigue, pain, and bladder dysfunction, that cause so much of the discomfort associated with MS.

Treating Exacerbations

When a person is experiencing an MS attack, the doctor's first priority is usually to stop the inflammation process. For many years the standard treatment has been to suppress the inflammatory activity of the immune system. This is effective in the short-term, but does not affect the long-term outcome of MS.

Adrenocorticotropic hormone (ACTH) and corticosteroids have been used for over thirty years to treat autoimmune conditions such as MS, lupus, and transplant rejection. In comparative studies, steroids such as prednisolone and methylprednisolone are slightly more effective than ACTH in preventing a relapse of MS. The intravenous administration of steroids appears to be more effective than oral administration. The use of steroids to stop inflammation has observable positive effects on the blood-brain barrier (as shown by MRIs), immunoglobulin levels, and other immunological markers.

The drawback of steroids is their cumulative side effects, which include stomach irritation, elevation of blood sugar, water retention, insomnia, and mood swings. Long courses of corticosteroids can suppress their natural production by the adrenal gland, so the dosage should be tapered when discontinuing use. For MS patients, the associated loss of bone density, which can lead to frequent fractures and osteoporosis, is of paramount concern. Therefore, doctors limit the duration and frequency of steroid usage on a case-by-case basis.

Disease-Modifying Treatments

Several therapies can delay the progression of certain types of MS (see table 4.1). These disease-modifying treatments increase the duration of time between attacks, increasing the ability of MS patients to recover between them. Treatment selection is determined by the type of MS a patient exhibits.

Avonex

Avonex is a synthetic version of a cytokine produced by human immune cells. The manufacturing process involves expression of the human gene for interferon beta-1a in Chinese hamster ovary cells. In healthy people, interferons regulate the immune response to viral infections and tumors. In MS, they decrease the migration of immune cells into the CNS, inhibit T cell proliferation, and signal the production of other cytokines that promote remyelination and axon repair.

Avonex is used to treat patients with relapsing forms of MS, and may be used in people who have had only a single attack if their MRI analysis also indicates features of MS. Avonex is administered weekly by intramuscular injection. Recipients of Avonex may experience flu-like symptoms after

Table 4.1 Comparison of Disease-Modifying Drugs

Brand Name	Generic Name	Manufacturer	Type of MS	Administration Method
Avonex	Interferon beta-1a	Biogen, Inc.	Relapsing	Weekly intramuscular injection
Betaseron	Interferon beta-1b	Berlex Labs, Inc.	Relapsing, including secondary progressive	Subcutaneous injection every other day
Copaxone	Glatiramer acetate	Teva Pharmaceutical Industries	Relapsing-remitting	Daily subcutaneous injection
Rebif	Interferon beta-1a	Serono, Inc.	Relapsing	Subcutaneous injection three times weekly
Novantrone	Mitoxantrone	Immunex	Rapidly worsening relapsing, progressive-relapsing, or secondary progressive	Four intravenous injections per year

an injection, but this side effect lessens with time for many people. More rare side effects include depression, anemia, liver damage, and allergic reactions.

Betaseron

Betaseron, or interferon beta-1b, differs from Avonex by one amino acid (amino acid 17 is changed from cysteine to serine). It also lacks the carbohydrate modification on amino acid 80, which Avonex has. Betaseron is produced by expression of its gene in bacteria. It is used to treat people with relapsing forms of MS and can even help those with secondary progressive MS if they still experience noticeable relapses.

Betaseron is administered every other day by subcutaneous injection. Common side effects of taking Betaseron include flu-like symptoms and injection site allergic reactions, some of which necessitate medical attention. Less common side effects include depression, elevated liver enzymes, and low white blood cell counts.

Copaxone

Glatiramer acetate, brand name Copaxone and formerly known as Copolymer-1, was originally designed to induce MS-like symptoms in animals. Its structure, random polymers of four amino acids (glutamic acid, lysine, alanine, and tyrosine, thus the name GLATiramer), was supposed to induce an autoimmune response by mimicking a protein found in myelin. Contrary to the expectation, it reduced the occurrence of symptoms in animals and was successful in later human trials that tested its effect on relapsing-remitting forms of MS.

Although its mechanism of action is not well defined, Copaxone is thought to activate anti-inflammatory T cells, which can inhibit local immune reactions within the CNS.

Copaxone is administered daily by subcutaneous injection. The most common side effect of this treatment is a mild allergic reaction at the injection site. Less common side effects include vasodilation, chest pain, and symptoms of anxiety, including heart palpitations, shortness of breath, and flushed skin. The less common side effects last about fifteen to thirty minutes and have no known long-term consequences.

Rebif

Rebif is an alternate form of interferon beta-1a. Its chemical composition is the same as Avonex, but it is administered with a different regimen. Rebif was first approved in Europe for treating relapsing forms of MS, and was approved by the FDA for distribution in the U.S. in 2002.

It is injected subcutaneously three times per week. The most common side effects are flu-like symptoms, which lessen with time for many patients, and allergic reactions at the injection site. Nausea can be alleviated in many people by a ramped dosage schedule, which allows the patient to become acclimated to the drug. (This is also true for Avonex and Betaseron.) Less common side effects include liver abnormalities, depression, and low red or white blood cell counts.

Novantrone

Novantrone, or mitoxantrone, is the newest disease-modifying therapeutic. The FDA approved it for manufacture and distribution by Immunex in 2002. Novantrone targets rapidly worsening relapsing-remitting MS and progressive relapsing or secondary progressive MS. Its mechanism of action is undefined, but it generally enhances the activity of immune suppressor cells and directly suppresses both T and B cells. It also appears to deactivate macrophages and induce the death of antigen-presenting cells. In clinical trials, it decreased the number of recurring attacks and slowed the rate of increasing disability.

Novantrone is administered by intravenous infusion four times a year in a medical facility. While it has potent effects that relieve MS symptoms, potentially serious side effects occur when a certain cumulative dosage is reached. It may cause heart failure, sterility, and birth defects, and some instances of leukemia have been linked to treatment with mitoxantrone. Because the dosage is limited by these side effects, particularly the cardiotoxicity, mitoxantrone can only be taken for a maximum of three years. The lifetime limit is eight to twelve doses, but the positive effects of this drug last for at least a year beyond the termination of treatment. Clinical studies continue to determine which types of MS respond best to mitoxantrone, and to investigate its side effect profile.

A person who takes Novantrone may not be allowed to use any of the other disease-modifying drugs. The current outlook is that it will be most useful as the initial therapy for people with very active forms of MS or as an alternative treatment for those whose symptoms do not respond to the interferons or glatiramer acetate.

Treatments for Specific Symptoms

No treatment has been shown to alter the course of MS over more than a decade, and eventually the MS patient will have to deal with the symptoms associated with the disease. Fortunately, there has been as much research on treating symptoms as there has been for disease modification, and there are many options for making life with MS more comfortable.

Vision Problems

Optic neuritis, the most common visual effect in MS, is the result of inflammatory activity in the immune system. It is therefore most often treated by administration of a corticosteroid such as prednisolone or methylprednisolone to stop the inflammation. This treatment is not indicated for long-term use and, while it may shorten the duration of the individual attack, has no demonstrated effect on the degree or duration of recovery.

Poor Coordination

Loss of coordination, or ataxia, and the tremors associated with it are among the hardest MS symptoms to treat. Isoniazid, carbamazepine, clonazepam, buspirone, and ondansetron have each been tested for their ability to lessen tremor. Several small studies have been done, all producing less than convincing results. Thalamotomy (removal of the ventral intermediate nucleus from the brain) has been shown to reduce tremor in Parkinson's disease, but has limited effectiveness for treating MS. Its drawbacks are its permanence, the lack of data on side effects, and the possibility that tremor will return in a short period of time.

Spasticity

Spasticity, a state of strong muscular contraction, can be the cause or the result of MS-associated pain. It is commonly the underlying cause of urinary incontinence. Management of spasticity often requires several strategies ranging from proper positioning of limbs to use of medications. Baclofen (Lioresal) and tizanidine (Zanaflex), the most common drugs for treating spasticity, are depressants that inhibit nerve signal transmission by binding to and activating a receptor that affects the balance of ions at neuronal termini. Dantrolene (Dantrium) acts directly on muscles to lessen the force of contractions, which may result in increasing weakness. For this reason, it is better suited to patients whose mobility is already limited. Clonazepam (Klonopin) is from a class of molecules called *benzodiazepines*, which act as anticonvulsants by binding to a receptor that inhibits neural activity in the brain. They suppress sensory impulses in both nerves and muscles. Gabapentin (Neurontin) is usually given as a supplementary treatment for more advanced cases of MS. Its mechanism of action is unknown, but it has the effect of an anticonvulsant. Botulinum A Toxin (Botox) is helpful for people with severe localized muscle spasms. It can reduce spasticity for up to three months by inhibiting the release of excitatory molecules at nerve junctions.

Pain

Pain is a secondary symptom—one that is caused by a primary symptom. Treatments for pain are tailored to the probable cause of the pain, such as muscle contractions, spasticity, or optic neuritis. The less specific pains are treated with drugs that affect the CNS in general, such as tricyclic antidepressants and anti-epileptic medications.

Tricyclic antidepressants are commonly used to treat MS pain. Some of the neural pathways controlling depression overlap with those controlling physical pain, which is why these work for both. These medications, including nortriptyline (Pamelor), amitriptyline (Elavil), and imipramine (Tofranil), block the uptake of serotonin by nerve cells, making more of this neurotransmitter available for stimulating nerve impulses. Tricyclic antidepressants enhance the drowsiness caused by alcohol and other CNS depressants, such as antihistamines and sleep medications. Other common side effects include dryness of the mouth, extreme sensitivity of the skin to sunlight, and increases in blood sugar levels. Withdrawal effects can be pronounced, so most doctors taper the prescribed dosage as a patient comes off these medications.

Anti-epileptic medications are also used to treat MS pain. These include phenytoin (Dilantin) and gabapentin (Neurontin), which are used to treat pain caused by abnormal sensory pathways in the CNS and spasticity, respectively. Phenytoin binds to sodium channels in the neuronal membrane and keeps them from conducting the ions necessary for nerve signal transmission. Gabapentin is thought to have the same effect by its binding to calcium channels. Like the tricyclic antidepressants, these medications can increase the drowsiness associated with alcohol or other medications. Use of antacids or diarrhea medicines can interfere with their effects and should be avoided within several hours of each dose.

Cognitive Dysfunction

Mental changes in people with MS can range from slight memory loss and slow learning to severe depression. There are no medications that improve memory or stimulate problem-solving ability, but depression can be treated medicinally with a variety of drugs. Tricyclic antidepressants are a major type of depression treatment, and as noted above, they are also used to treat some types of pain. Based on the success of these stimulants, other drugs have been designed to do the same thing. Examples are paroxetine (Paxil), fluoxetine hydrochloride (Prozac), and sertraline (Zoloft). Because of their stimulant status, these drugs may interfere with attempts to treat spasticity, the aim of which is to block nerve signal transmission.

Fatigue

Since fatigue has many causes, both physical and psychological, there are many possible ways to treat it. A regular exercise regimen, for example, improves daily performance of routine tasks. Also, the mental stressors that trigger fatigue can be lessened by simply avoiding overexposure to stressful situations, social or otherwise. For more persistent physical symptoms of fatigue, amantadine (Symmetrel), an anti-viral compound used to treat certain flu infections, has been shown to be useful, though its mechanism is unknown. A daily dose of 100–200 milligrams is taken before noon. Side effects unique to amantadine include dryness of the mouth and possible dark blotchy marks on the skin, usually on the lower legs. Modafinil (Provigil) is a CNS stimulant that promotes wakefulness. It can also cause general changes in mood, perception, and thinking abilities. A daily dose of 100–200 milligrams is taken early in the day, with higher doses having less effect. This drug has been approved in the U.S. for treatment of narcolepsy, not MS, so the known side effects have been gleaned from studies of that condition. Pemoline (Cylert) is used to treat attention deficit disorders and is sometimes tried for MS-related fatigue, though at least one study found that it had no greater effect than a placebo. Anywhere from 20–140 milligrams per day is taken before mid-afternoon to avoid sleep disturbances. Pemoline makes some people feel dizzy or less alert, and its manufacturers and the FDA suggest biweekly checks of liver function of patients taking the drug.

Bladder and Bowel Problems

Tolterodine (Detrol) and oxybutinin (Ditropan) are used to control bladder spasms that cause urinary frequency or incontinence. Oxybutinin is available as an extended-release pill that can be taken once a day or as a skin patch that is applied twice weekly. Other medications that treat urinary frequency or incontinence are propantheline (Pro-Banthine) and imipramine (Tofranil). Desmopressin is a synthetic version of the naturally occurring antidiuretic hormone that controls urinary frequency by temporarily blocking the production of urine. It is available as either a nasal spray (DDAVP Nasal Spray) or a tablet (DDAVP Tablets).

For constipation the main treatment is some type of laxative, which can usually be purchased without a prescription. Different laxatives have different side effects and work in different ways and on different time scales. Some are available in different forms: as tablets, granules, or suppositories. No laxative is meant to be a long-term treatment, and each is most effective when used in conjunction with other strategies that promote healthy bowel function, such as a well-balanced diet and a regular exercise regimen.

A hyperosmotic laxative uses high salt concentrations to draw water into the intestines and promote bowel movements.

Magnesium hydroxide (Milk of Magnesia) is the most common one, but suppositories containing glycerin (Sani-Supp suppository) produce the same effect in the same way. A stool softener helps liquids mix into solid stool so it is more easily passed through the bowels. Docusate (Colace) is an example of this type. Stimulant laxatives are the most popular, but they have the most side effects. Bisacodyl (Dulcolax) increases the muscle contractions of the large intestine so that stool is passed more easily. Mineral oil is a lubricant laxative. It coats the bowel and the stool, which helps to retain the moisture necessary for easy passage. Psyllium hydrophilic mucilloid (Metamucil) is a bulk-forming laxative. It is not absorbed by the body, but swells in the intestines to form a stool that stimulates normal passage of fecal material.

Sexual Dysfunction

Sexual dysfunction has both psychological and physiological aspects, and the distinction between the two is poorly understood. Current studies have addressed only the physiology of erectile dysfunction, and the treatments available for MS are the same as those for the general public. Sildenafil citrate (Viagra) helps maintain penile erection by delaying the activity of phosphodiesterases, enzymes that degrade a molecule called cyclic guanine monophosphate (GMP). Cyclic GMP relaxes smooth muscle in the penis, which enhances the inflow of blood that creates an erection. Several new analogs of sildenafil have recently been introduced, but they have not been tested in MS patients. The effects of sildenafil on the sexual functioning of women with spinal cord injury have been studied, and the results suggest it increases arousal.

Alternative Treatments

Up to 75 percent of people with MS use complementary or alternative medicine to treat their symptoms. Complementary medicine is that which is taken in addition to medically approved treatments, whereas alternative medicine is used in place of those treatments. The difference is that conventional medicine has been shown to be safe and effective. The claims of alternative medicine are not backed by experimental evidence. Nonprescription treatments for MS may interact with standard therapy, and accurate records of the dosage schedule are needed to correlate any changes in overall health with the supplemental treatment.

Vitamins

Vitamins are normally obtained from the diet, sometimes supplemented by a pill. Vitamin D is the only vitamin that humans can synthesize, and that occurs during exposure of the skin to sunlight. It is possible that the geographic distribution of MS incidence is related to reduced sun exposure in the northern hemisphere during the winter months. Across different populations, MS exacerbations are more common in the spring. Some studies suggest a lag time of two months between the winter drop in vitamin D levels and the onset of MS symptoms.

Munger and co-workers at Harvard's Department of Nutrition recently reported the results of a large study that demonstrated a correlation between vitamin D intake and MS. Over ten to twenty years, women with high vitamin D intake were 40 percent less likely to have MS. All women in the upper quintile of vitamin D levels were taking supplements, and there was no additional benefit afforded by vitamin D obtained from the diet. Nutrition experts agree that the current recommended daily amount of vitamin D is insufficient even to maintain bone density, so supplementation for all people (not just those with MS or at risk for MS) is recommended.

Vitamin D levels correlate with several autoimmune diseases in addition to MS: rheumatoid arthritis, inflammatory bowel disease, and insulin-dependent (type 2) diabetes mellitus. This essential vitamin appears to alter the balance of T cell populations, promoting the proliferation of regulatory T cells that keep inflammation in check. Low levels of vitamin D result in abnormally high numbers of pro-inflammatory T cells, which favors the onset of autoimmune conditions. Vitamin D also helps to prevent osteoporosis, to which people with MS are susceptible due to decreased physical activity and steroid treatments.

CNS inflammation releases reactive oxygen species, which are highly reactive molecules containing an unpaired electron. Reactive oxygen species can damage cellular building blocks such as myelin and DNA. Vitamins A, C, and E are known antioxidants, compounds that fight the damage caused by reactive oxygen species. These vitamins might help prevent or reduce the effects of inflammatory demyelination. Vitamin C is also used as a preventive measure against urinary tract infections. This effect is unproven, and there are other treatments that may work more effectively.

Vitamin B_{12} helps produce red blood cells and assists in proper functioning of the nervous system. Vitamin B_{12} deficiency produces neurological symptoms similar to MS. It is worthwhile to be tested for B_{12} levels and to take a vitamin supplement if they are discovered to be lower than normal.

Minerals

Minerals are essential elements that our bodies do not manufacture on their own. Some studies have shown that people with MS may have slightly lower levels of selenium, an antioxidant mineral. There are conflicting reports about the effects of selenium on MS, and selenium may actually increase the immune response, so selenium supplements, if used, should be used in moderation.

Calcium is the most abundant mineral in the body. It plays a fundamental role in biology, acting in processes as diverse as muscle contraction, cell signaling, and nerve stimulation. It is also essential for building and maintaining strong bones. Its main benefit in people with MS is to prevent osteoporosis. Adequate vitamin D intake is essential for proper absorption of calcium.

Herbs

Herbs used as alternatives to conventional therapies are whole plants or parts of plants that may contain many different substances mixed together. Because they are not pure preparations of a single compound, they may produce different effects in different people and should be used with caution. Moreover, their production and labeling are not regulated in the way that prescription drugs are.

Ginkgo biloba is a popular herb said to enhance cognitive function. It is known to inhibit blood clotting. Several studies of the effects of this herb on exacerbations in people with MS have shown either a small positive effect or no effect at all. Its effects on cognitive function are as yet untested.

Echinacea is often used to treat the common cold. While support of the medical community for this strategy is partially positive, echinacea may stimulate the immune system. For this reason, people with MS should avoid echinacea.

St. John's wort has been used to treat depression. However, a large and definitive study concluded in 2002 demonstrated that this herb has no benefit in treating depression compared with placebos. On the other hand, no studies have suggested that St. John's wort is actually harmful to MS patients, and the jury is still out on whether it helps people with minor feelings of depression. St. John's wort interacts with a variety of drugs and metabolic processes, so caution should be exercised in deciding to take it.

Valerian has been proven effective in helping people fall asleep faster. However, its effects on the immune system are not known. People who have fatigue should be careful about valerian, since it may produce lingering sedative effects.

Cranberry juice can prevent urinary tract infections. It prevents bacteria from adhering to the epithelial cells that line the urinary tract. It should not, however, be used to treat an existing infection, which instead requires a course of antibiotics.

5. Living with MS

Everything changes after a diagnosis with MS. Coping with the news requires mental and emotional adjustments of greater proportion than almost any other life event. This chapter discusses ways of handling the initial emotions, mechanisms for coping with a chronic illness like MS, and concerns about relationships with family members and friends. Recommendations for lifestyle choices and financial planning round out this primer on living with MS.

Mental and Emotional Adjustments

A diagnosis with multiple sclerosis affects every part of a person's life. Common initial reactions include denial, anger, fear, grief, depression, and guilt. It is normal to feel that the situation is unfair or unbearable. Denial can actually protect an individual from experiencing the more negative emotions and is considered healthy as long as it does not interfere with making decisions about treatment. Grief is also a health-promoting reaction when allowed to run its course. Mourning for the loss of past health and independence is essential to letting go and facing the future. As MS progresses, emotional changes should be expected and dealt with as they arise.

People with MS have a particularly difficult task: learning to cope with uncertainty. Because the cause of MS is not known, they often wonder if they did something to "deserve" it. Even the diagnosis may have been a long process because of the sporadic occurrence of symptoms. The unpredictability of symptoms adds to the frustration of increasing or impending immobility, and fear of an unpredictable future heightens stress. Flexibility and optimism are positive character traits to develop in dealing with a relapsing-remitting chronic illness. Learning to accept change with hope is helpful in adjusting to new situations successfully.

The connection between the mind and the body is well established. A positive outlook has many health benefits, including reduced stress, less anxiety, and fewer illnesses. Realistic expectations of people and situations alleviate mood swings. Staying involved in the world at large provides much-needed respite from constantly dealing with decisions about handling MS. A fundamental component of mental health for many people is spirituality. Faith and prayer can be powerful tools for coping, and attendance at religious services has been correlated with the ability to successfully handle chronic illness.

Strategic Coping Mechanisms

Because MS affects each individual differently, coping strategies vary from person to person. Finding the right combination of strategies is important for maintaining independence. The goal should be to differentiate between which situations can be controlled and which cannot, and to maintain as much control as possible. Flexibility is key to adapting to life with MS.

Education is one of the most powerful ways to deal with the uncertainty that characterizes MS. Understanding the basic science removes the guilt-based suspicion that personal behavior somehow triggered the disease. A solid knowledge base also bolsters confidence when answering questions about MS from friends and family members. Staying abreast of ongoing research prepares the patient to make informed decisions when new treatments emerge. Detailed information about assistive devices is beneficial in managing symptoms.

Building a support system is crucial to coping successfully with MS. Open communication about emotions, both positive and negative, strengthens families to survive the inevitable changes in activities and responsibilities. An atmosphere of empathy and support brings family members closer together. Investing time in established friendships helps to retain some normalcy during times of drastic change. Friends who have some distance from the MS embody a valuable connection to the "outside" world. An MS support group is also beneficial, providing a feeling of community with people who share the same situation. It is also a convenient resource for practical ideas about handling everyday concerns. One-on-one counseling can also be of assistance to some people.

Self-advocacy at the doctor's office is another important mechanism for coping with MS. When dealing with physicians, it is essential to find a balance between being assertive and listening to the advice of experts. Initiating discussion of symptoms and treatments shows that the patient is reasonably well informed and ready to make decisions. Open dialogue is facilitated by preparing questions in advance, keeping an accurate and up-to-date diary of symptoms, and taking notes during the discussion. Self-education is essential for both self-expression and comprehension of the doctor's directives. Knowing why a certain treatment or no treatment is recommended is important to peace of mind, as is the ability to decline treatment suggestions that do not feel right.

One way to stay involved in society is to participate in government affairs, and people with chronic illnesses have a personal motivation to do so. Many legislative decisions affect people with chronic illnesses or disabilities. Congressional representatives need to hear from their constituents on issues such as federally funded research, health insurance laws, long-term health care, and rights for disabled people. Staying informed on these issues requires reading from a variety of news sources. The National Multiple Sclerosis Society website (www.nmss.org/advocacy.asp) collates pertinent legislative information in one convenient location so that interested readers can participate effectively as political advocates.

A connection with the working world helps some people with MS maintain a sense of independence. Additional benefits include meaningful social interaction and, obviously, income. However, many people with MS experience substantial angst over the possible effects of MS on their jobs. When obtaining or keeping employment, the question of disclosure is foremost: who should be told about the MS, in what way, and in how much detail? Expert advice from a counselor is extremely helpful in making the decision to tell, and planning ahead what to say and how to say it will make the disclosure less uncomfortable. Several factors increase the viability of employment for people with MS. First, knowledge of the basic science of MS helps in explaining to others what MS is and how it affects those who have it. Answering questions from bosses and co-workers sets their minds at ease and reduces the tendency toward negative assumptions. Second, familiarity with the provisions of the Americans with Disabilities Act will instill confidence to request accommodations in scheduling, duties, or facilities when needed. It is up to the individual with MS to initiate discussion of accommodations; this is best done before a crisis occurs. Most employers are knowledgeable about the law and are willing to respond to employees whose goal is increased productivity. Finally, it is important to be realistic about the viability of employment. If leaving the workplace becomes necessary, planning for alternative sources of income and insurance eases the transition. At the same time, exiting the work force prematurely because of unfounded fears is unnecessary, and expert advice on setting realistic expectations is extremely helpful.

Relationships

A diagnosis with MS changes every relationship in a person's life. Spouses, children, parents, siblings, and friends are likely to react in different ways, each experiencing a range of emotions similar to those felt by the individual with MS. Because each individual will handle the situation differently, there are no definite guidelines for how to deal with the chronic illness of a loved one. One of the most helpful coping mechanisms is reading or listening to someone else's experience of the same thing, which alleviates loneliness and provides some general patterns to apply.

Spouses have a unique challenge in coping with the diagnosis of their life partner with MS and the impending changes that accompany it. In addition to initial reactions of anger or fear, spouses often deal with heightened feelings of disappointment, guilt, and loneliness. For spouses who become the primary caregiver, the perception of abandonment by friends and family is a common experience. Obtaining support from any and all available sources is essential to the survival of the marriage and to the health of the well spouse. People who cope successfully with the chronic illness of their partner implement several common strategies. First, they learn to ask for help. Relatives, friends, health-care professionals, and counselors all represent resources for physical or emotional support, and the well spouse learns to combine the assistance offered from each of these relationships. The well spouse must also adjust his or her expectations of roles within the relationship. MS may cause sudden changes in physical abilities that require the well spouse to be both homemaker and breadwinner, both caregiver and sexual partner, in ways that have not been experienced before. Adjustment to new routines and new plans is also required. Daily, weekly, and monthly activities may have to be modified on short notice, and long-term plans for retirement or travel may require alteration. A well spouse should maintain some degree of independence, both physically and mentally. For a spouse who is the primary caregiver, time away from home is essential for reviving the spirit. Social connections help maintain perspective and provide much needed support. Pursuit of personal interests keeps the body healthy and the mind sharp. Finally, well spouses must learn to share their feelings openly, tactfully, but without guilt. Both spouses can be expected to experience a full range of emotions, since both are feeling the pain of MS in different ways. Support groups or couples' counseling sessions may help to achieve the openness required to maintain a healthy marriage against the background of a chronic illness such as MS.

Children of people with MS have special concerns about the uncertainty of the disease. Younger children may have trouble understanding exactly what MS means to them, and they may experience irritation over the shift in attention from themselves to the parent with MS. They need reassurance that while things might change at a physical level, the family bond and its structure will remain intact. Older children might be afraid of what their friends will think or how MS will affect their responsibilities at home. Teaching them about the basic facts of MS will equip them to answer questions from their friends, and careful distribution of extra chores should prevent them from shouldering too much responsibility. Children of any age should not be given the task of primary caregiving, since the emotional and mental tolls of this role are great. Teenagers can expect increased responsibility at home compared with their peers who have well parents. Feelings of guilt for neglecting a sick parent, anxiety over financial status, or embarrassment over a parent's disability are all normal. Helpful coping strategies include keeping a journal, communicating about feelings, getting a job, and keeping outside friendships alive. These activities can alleviate tension at home and promote feelings of independence without guilt.

Extended family members also experience a range of emotional and mental reactions to the news of a diagnosis with MS. Often, they would like to offer help but hesitate to do so. They might feel like intruders in a private situation, or they might be doubtful about how much help they can actually provide. Family and friends who want to lend support should be welcomed whenever possible, and clear communication about the needs of the person with MS can relieve uncertainties of both parties. Different people have different types of assistance to offer, so it is expedient to have several options among which they can choose. Some might like to provide carpool and child-care services, while others would enjoy preparing a meal or two. Another way to make people feel comfortable offering help is to define their commitment. For instance, asking them to babysit for three hours on a Saturday while the spouse runs errands or does housework sets specific limits on their time and helps them plan the rest of their day. This type of exchange prevents unmet expectations and allows people to offer help at their convenience.

Friends of the family affected by MS can help keep them connected to the outside world. Unfortunately, friendships cannot always withstand the pressure of the changes MS brings. The energy level and physical abilities of the friend with MS may require significant alterations in the locales and scheduling of social activities. Friendships can seem one-sided or guilt-based rather than mutual and voluntary, but are essential to keep life from revolving around MS twenty-four hours a day. Work to keep communication open. Well friends do not want to feel tied down, and the person with MS does not want to feel left behind. Time together may have to be more limited than before, and each party should say plainly what works for them. Even if past friendships dissolve, new ones may develop with others who share the experience of life with MS. Friendships between individuals with MS and their families provide a unique kind of support, camaraderie, and encouragement.

The caregiver balances independence and assistance for the person with MS. Most often, the primary caregiver is a spouse, but it can also be a family member or hired professional. This person assists with anything and everything, from basic household tasks like cleaning and laundry to intimate personal care such as showering and using the bathroom. The close contact required for some of these duties increases the need for independence in other areas of life, especially if the caregiver is a spouse or a live-in family member. Caregiving requires time, energy, and commitment, and caregivers need mental and social outlets to refresh their spirits. Caregivers who are hired can view caregiving as a job with limited demands on their time; however, live-in caregivers whose waking hours are devoted primarily to caregiving need special consideration. Time off should be arranged on a regular basis, whether for a few hours or a whole day or more. With spousal caregivers, there is potential for self-neglect, usually rooted in guilt about being healthy. Wives who care for their husbands with MS are particularly prone to neglecting their own health or personal development. This eventually produces resentment in both the caregiver and the person with MS, leading to increased probability of verbal or physical abuse. Counseling with someone who specializes in dealing with the issues raised by chronic illness can help solve these problems. Finding support from other couples who have experienced the same frustrations is also helpful. Coping with the situation requires making a specific plan for living that meets the needs of both partners by taking into account their differences in abilities, energy levels, and personal preferences.

Lifestyle

"Eat right and exercise." This directive is repeated by dietitians, weight-loss professionals, and personal trainers. It is the key to staying healthy, maintaining weight, and increasing longevity, and it applies to everyone, including people with MS.

The nutritional needs of people with MS are basically the same as for anyone. Whole grains, fruits, vegetables, and low-fat proteins should constitute the majority of each day's menu. Medications can affect appetite and metabolism and may require adjustments in the amounts and combinations of foods eaten, as well as in the level of activity required to maintain a healthy weight.

In addition to eating healthfully, an exercise routine should be established. The recommendation for people in good health is thirty to forty minutes of cardiovascular and/or muscular work at least three times per week. People with MS can adhere to this guideline when their symptoms permit. However, during and following an exacerbation, or after the MS progresses to the point of physical disability, the duration and type of exercise should be tailored to the individual's abilities.

In deciding what type of exercise to do, special considerations should be made for personal preferences and physical limitations. People with MS are especially prone to overworking when their symptoms are in remission, but this can backfire and cause symptoms to reappear or worsen. Overheating can also exacerbate MS symptoms and should be carefully avoided. Some people prefer solo exercise to a group setting, in which case walking, jogging, and biking are good choices. Tennis or other sports are good for those who enjoy company while exercising. Swimming is a very popular exercise among people with MS because it prevents overheating and because movement of limbs is easier in the water. As with any exercise regimen, stretching is an important part of warming up and cooling down and also prevents injury to spastic muscles.

One of the most difficult adjustments to MS is the loss of physical fitness during exacerbations. Returning to the previous level of activity can be challenging and time-consuming. Patience, realistic expectations, and open-mindedness can ease this transition time. A few minutes of activity is better than none at all, and overworking can result in regression rather than progress in physical fitness. Some people may have to adjust their workout to contain more muscular work and less cardiovascular work at first. Strength is essential for regaining bodily control after an exacerbation, and is at least as important as cardiovascular fitness during the initial recovery period. In some cases, physical therapy may be required to teach the body how to move properly again. If there is a permanent loss of function, new exercise methods and schedules should be arranged.

Physical Aids

The time eventually comes when most people with MS need physical assistance with routine tasks. Help can be provided by another person, but to maintain some degree of independence many people prefer to use assistive devices. These include everything from small handles for gripping pens and pencils to motorized wheelchairs and custom-designed home modifications. While using any of these devices requires adjustment, the independence they offer is liberating to most people.

There are several potential barriers to using an assistive device. Anxiety over the perception of others may inhibit a person from using a cane or a walker in public. This fear should be weighed against the possibility of a fall, which would undoubtedly cause embarrassment and possibly also result in injury. Learning to use a new piece of equipment can consume a lot of energy, something that people with MS do not have to spare. Patience, planning, and persistence will help smooth the transition to a new way of doing things. Finally, the cost of electronic devices or large-scale home modifications can be prohibitive. In this case, filing an insurance claim or locating a charity that provides specific devices can defray some of the costs of making life with MS a little easier.

The Internet contains a wealth of information on assistive devices. Offerings range from devices providing assistance with daily activities such as eating, bathing, and dressing to those that ease the transition from home to work, school, or other environments. Specialized equipment is available for performing such tasks as dialing the telephone, using a computer, and driving. Participation in sporting activities is also covered, as are basic transportation needs. A physical or occupational therapist can give advice on what devices to use in specific situations. The wide variety of options is a reminder that many physical limitations can be overcome with a little creative thinking.

Planning for the Future

Coping with MS involves planning for an uncertain future. It is important to gather as much information as possible about health insurance, long-term care, and treatment options. Family and financial planning will depend greatly on the rate and degree of progression of MS. A balance of realism and optimism can make decisions in these areas more manageable.

Health insurance can be obtained through an employer, an individual policy, or from the government. Laws governing the availability and cost of health insurance differ from state to state. Health insurance consumer guides are available from each state and contain information about the process of obtaining insurance, different types of private insurance coverage, and state-funded insurance programs. Medicare is the federal program providing health insurance to those who qualify. Regardless of age or income, people with MS are eligible for Medicare once they have received twenty-four months of Social Security disability benefits. Recent changes in Medicare benefits include coverage of a limited number of people with MS for treatment with disease-modifying therapies and availability of drug discount cards that offer up to 50 percent savings for certain generic prescription drugs.

Financial planning should take into account the possible need for long-term care. Priority should be given to saving and investing; outstanding debt should be minimized. Long-term care is only partly covered by Medicare, with the remaining costs falling on the family of the MS patient. Also, plans to start or expand the family may have to be modified with regard to timing or extent. Changes in financial status or physical condition can affect the ability to raise children. Outside assistance from friends and family works well temporarily, but long-term financial plans should account for the future needs of each family member.

Another form of insurance against an uncertain future is the use of advance medical directives. Such directives ensure that the health-care preferences of MS patients are known and followed should they ever become incapable of expressing those preferences. A living will informs physicians of the desired emergency or long-term treatments. A health-care proxy may be appointed by granting power of attorney to a trusted relative or friend. Either of these measures ensures that health-care providers are legally bound to comply with the wishes of the person with MS. Laws governing health-care planning vary by state of residence, and an attorney can help navigate the choices.

6. The Search for a Cure

The number of clinical trials of MS drugs has increased rapidly over the last decade. With the success of the interferons and glatiramer acetate, researchers have been motivated to look for additional treatments. Several new drugs are in clinical trials, and much basic research is being done to produce the next generation of therapies. New treatments under investigation target various aspects of MS pathogenesis, from migration of immune cells into the CNS to proliferation of immune cells during inflammation and neuronal degeneration resulting from repeated demyelination. The research outlook for MS is increasingly promising as time, effort, and funds are directed toward the search for a cure.

The Clinical Trials Process

To be approved as an MS treatment, a drug must pass through three phases of clinical trials. Phase I trials determine the safety of a drug in humans. Usually, a small number of healthy volunteers are paid to participate in a study that lasts for several months. If the drug is not too toxic, researchers proceed with phase II trials, which are designed to determine the appropriate dosage. These trials include real patients for whom the drug was developed and are usually double-blinded, meaning that neither the researchers nor the patients know if they are receiving the active drug or a placebo. Phase II trials last up to two years. Phase III clinical trials observe the effects of the drug in thousands of patients over several years. These trials establish efficacy of the drug, sometimes in direct comparison with an existing treatment, and profile its side effects. Even after approval of a drug, ongoing studies continue to evaluate its long-term efficacy and side effects.

People interested in participating in clinical trials should consult their doctor, who should be able to refer them to studies for which they are eligible. Alternatively, the National MS Society or the North American Research Consortium on MS can provide information on trials open for recruitment. ClinicalTrials.gov, a website sponsored by the National Institutes of Health, is another online resource for locating clinical trials. To be accepted for a trial, patients must meet eligibility requirements in the areas of age, sex, type of MS, level of disability, and prior treatments. Once accepted, the patient should become well informed about the purposes, potential risks, and potential benefits of participation. Even after being accepted, the patient is free to leave a trial at any time for any reason. Participating in a clinical trial allows a person access to the latest treatments (even before they become generally available) under expert medical care at the top facilities in their area. Clinical trial volunteers also have the satisfaction of contributing to gains in medical understanding.

Emerging Treatments

MS pathogenesis is characterized by an initial inflammatory phase, followed by demyelination and, finally, a neurodegenerative phase. New treatments for MS are directed mostly toward preventing CNS inflammation. The hope is that if inflammation can be stopped, demyelination can be delayed and neurodegeneration prevented.

Natalizumab

Antibodies that bind selectively to a single target molecule can be generated in the laboratory. Interaction between an antibody and its target can be used to prevent the target molecule from performing its biological function. Natalizumab is an antibody that binds to a cellular adhesion molecule (CAM) called very late antigen 4 (VLA 4). VLA 4 is an integrin that is expressed on the surface of activated leukocytes and mediates their adhesion to the blood-brain barrier. The binding of natalizumab to VLA 4 prevents VLA 4 from mediating migration of immune cells into the brain.

Natalizumab was successful in phase II clinical trials conducted by the International Natalizumab Multiple Sclerosis Trial Group, which includes researchers from the Institute of Neurology, London; Wayne State University School of Medicine, Detroit; the University of Miami School of Medicine, Miami; University Hospital, Nottingham, United Kingdom; the London Multiple Sclerosis Clinic, London, Ontario, Canada; Elan Pharmaceuticals, San Francisco; and St. Michael's Hospital, University of Toronto, Toronto. In this trial, treatment with natalizumab for six months decreased the number of new brain lesions in patients with relapsing-remitting or secondary progressive MS. Phase III clinical trials of natalizumab as an isolated treatment and a combination therapy are currently under way.

Other strategies for blocking the activity of CAMs include altering their expression within the parent cell and inhibiting the signaling pathways they trigger. Inhibition of CAMs is accomplished not only by antibodies but also by small molecules, which have the advantage of being less expensive to produce and less likely to trigger immune responses. Current research is comparing the benefits of targeting single CAMs versus entire families of CAMs. Because there is overlap of function among CAMs, the latter strategy may be more effective in stopping cell adhesion during inflammation.

Statins

Statins are a class of small molecules used to lower cholesterol, and they have recently been shown to possess immunomodulatory effects. Statins may modulate the immune system in several ways: inhibiting adhesion molecules, blocking synthesis of HLA molecules, or decreasing T cell proliferation. Further research is needed to determine exactly how statins work in MS patients.

Statins lessen the severity of experimental autoimmune encephalitis (EAE) in animals, and have been studied in small groups of humans. In preclinical studies at Karl-Franzens-Universitat in Graz, Austria, Oliver Neuhaus and co-workers showed that statins decrease the proliferation of lymphocytes isolated from people with MS and reduce the expression of adhesion molecules on the surface of T cells. In a recent clinical trial of simvastatin conducted by Timothy Vollmer and co-workers at the Barrow Neurological Institute of St. Joseph's Hospital and Medical Center in Phoenix, Arizona, people with relapsing-remitting MS exhibited a decrease in the number of new lesions appearing during the six-month treatment period. This result is considered preliminary, but the outlook for statins is generally very good because of the ease of administration (oral doses versus injections) and their safety record.

Estrogen

Because of the observation that MS exacerbations decrease during the final trimester of pregnancy and increase shortly after delivery, it is believed that estrogens may moderate the disease process. In mice, administration of estrogen reduces the secretion of inflammatory cytokines from activated T cells. Preclinical studies conducted in the laboratory of Rhonda Voskuhl at the UCLA Reed Neurological Research Center tested the effects of the pregnancy hormone estriol in nonpregnant women with MS. The subjects demonstrated a decrease in the number and size of brain lesions during six months of treatment with oral estriol. This effect was reversed when treatment ceased and returned when treatment was resumed six months later. In addition, the researchers observed a decrease in production of inflammatory cytokines and an increase in production of anti-inflammatory cytokines during the course of treatment.

Treatment with estriol and other estrogens requires further investigation, since it has been demonstrated that oral contraceptives, which contain estrogens, do not delay the onset of MS. Nevertheless, estrogens definitely allay the symptoms of several autoimmune diseases, including MS, rheumatoid arthritis, and psoriasis. Elucidation of the mechanisms by which estrogens mediate the immune response will potentially be applicable to more than one disease.

New Research Strategies

While the drugs discussed above are progressing through the clinical trial pipeline, new basic research is being done to produce the next generation of treatments. Recent advances in several areas have generated excitement within the MS research community. Armed with new information, researchers hope to discover new ways to diagnose and treat MS.

Genetic Analysis

DNA—deoxyribonucleic acid—is composed of chemical units called nucleotides. The entire set of DNA in a human cell is called the genome, and genes are discrete segments of DNA that encode single proteins or protein isoforms. The sequence of nucleotide units in a gene determines the identity of the proteins that are synthesized from that gene.

One way to study the genetic contribution to MS is to select a gene that encodes a protein known to function in MS pathogenesis, such as tumor necrosis factor or an intercellular adhesion protein, and study its sequence variation between different population groups. If the gene is associated with the onset of MS, people with MS might carry a certain allele more often than the general population. The drawback to this method is that a lot of time may be invested only to find out that the gene of interest is not very strongly associated with MS risk.

Determining the sequence of the entire human genome has allowed scientists to analyze genetic variation with a much broader view. The human genome has yielded insight into the baseline level of variability in certain chromosomes across different races and populations. In particular, it revealed specific regions of baseline variability within the human leukocyte antigen (HLA) genes, the only genes conclusively shown to be associated with MS. The sequences in these variable regions have no association with MS risk, and can, in the future, be excluded from consideration during genetic studies. Researchers can instead focus on regions of the HLA genes that might give insight into which alleles confer an increased risk of MS.

Research into the genetics of other neurological disorders has also shed light on the underlying mechanisms of MS. Charcot-Marie-Tooth disease (CMT) is a common genetic disorder of the peripheral nervous system. CMT is caused by duplication of a gene that encodes a myelin protein, PMP22. The gene exhibits a dosage effect in that a single copy gives rise to mild neuropathic symptoms, whereas four copies of the gene produce the more severe Dejerine-Sottas syndrome. This dosage effect is seen for certain MS-related HLA alleles, particularly the one designated DRB1*1501. People who have MS are more than twice as likely as the general population to possess this allele. Those with mild MS have only one copy, but people with severe forms of MS often have two copies. Future studies of dosage effects will benefit from separation of patients into subgroups based on disease subtypes. Researchers can then more easily identify alleles that affect the specific course of MS.

MS is a disease with complex inheritance characteristics, and leaders in the field acknowledge the need for larger genetic data sets from which to make statistically relevant comparisons. International collaborations will be necessary to gather and analyze genetic data from MS patients. One such collaboration is the HapMap project, in which scientists and funding agencies from Japan, the United Kingdom, Canada, China, Nigeria, and the United States are teaming up to determine the common polymorphisms within several different world populations. HapMap stands for haplotype mapping. Single nucleotide polymorphisms (SNPs) are often linked, and chromosomal regions that contain the same pattern of SNPs are called haplotypes. In the near future, MS researchers will be able to access the HapMap database, identify the haplotypes common to people with MS, and use the information to locate regions of the genome that are associated with MS.

The genetic causes of MS are complex, involving interactions between multiple polymorphic genes or groups of genes. Learning more about the genes that are linked to MS susceptibility will reveal specific mechanisms of disease onset and progression. Understanding the underlying mechanisms of MS will lead to new treatments for symptoms and eventually to therapies that will slow down or reverse the effects of MS. Until then, knowing the genetic basis of MS will help ensure accurate diagnosis and prognosis of the disease.

Microarray Analysis

Like people, cells have a defined life span. They are born, they grow and reproduce, and they die. At each stage of the cell cycle, different sets of genes are expressed, that is, they are used to produce proteins that determine the properties of the cell. Many of the approximately thirty thousand human genes have unknown functions, and the timing of gene expression is one indication of what their functions might be. For example, genes involved in cell division would be expressed just before cells divide.

Gene expression involves the synthesis of proteins using the DNA sequence as a template. One gene can be used to make thousands of copies of a protein, and this amplification occurs through an intermediate step involving synthesis of ribonucleic acid (RNA). RNA is chemically complementary to its parent DNA—that is, it can interact with that DNA via hydrogen bonding. RNA levels are indicative of how strongly a gene is being expressed, which in turn is a function of cell type and the stage of the cell cycle. Gene expression is altered during the course of a disease and can be used as a diagnostic tool.

Microarray analysis was developed in the 1990s as a way to detect the timing and levels of gene expression in different cells under various conditions. A microarray consists of a solid support chip or glass plate to which thousands of gene

Each position represents a
different gene sequence.

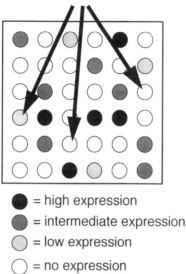

● = high expression

● = intermediate expression

◍ = low expression

○ = no expression

Figure 6.1 Microarray analysis. The position of the signal indicates which genes are being expressed. The intensity of the signal indicates how much RNA is being expressed by a particular gene, or to what extent it is "turned on"

fragments are attached (see fig. 6.1). Millions of DNA molecules can be attached to a chip that spans a few square inches, which is the reason the technique is considered "micro" in scale. The gene fragments are ordered in a linear array, with defined locations on the chip.

RNA is isolated from cells of a desired type and given time to interact with the DNA on the chip. The RNA interacts only with complementary DNA—that from which it was expressed. Non-interacting RNA is washed away, and bound RNA is visualized via a fluorescent molecule added to it during the isolation step. The strength of the fluorescence signal is directly proportional to the number of RNA molecules bound and is used to quantitate how much RNA was expressed from each gene in the cells. The position of the signal on the plate tells which genes were being expressed at the precise time the cell's RNA was isolated.

Microarray technology has been applied to cells within MS plaques obtained during autopsies. Not surprisingly, several studies found that genes involved in immune function, cell adhesion, and myelin production were being expressed. Genes implicated by this method represent targets for further study on their role in demyelination and axonal degeneration. Interestingly, comparisons between different types of MS plaques confirmed that the expression patterns in actively demyelinating plaques are different from those of silent plaques, which have expression patterns similar to healthy brain tissue.

In a collaboration between researchers at the Department of Neurology at Harvard Medical School and the Department of Chemical Engineering at Massachusetts Institute of Technology, Antonio Iglesias and co-workers used microarray analysis to study gene expression of peripheral blood mononuclear cells from MS patients. They found that interferon-responsive genes expressed in untreated patients returned to baseline levels in Avonex-treated patients. Thus, microarray analysis can be used to monitor the effects of different MS treatments. They also reported that the pattern of gene expression in MS patients was distinct from that of lupus patients, suggesting that microarray analysis can be used as a diagnostic tool to distinguish between neurological diseases and perhaps even disease subtypes. Finally, they detected activation of immune cells as indicated by increased expression of pro-inflammatory cytokine genes. Expression of these genes is dependent on a specific protein known as E2F1. When E2F1 was deleted from experimental mice in subsequent studies, the animals exhibited a less severe form of experimental auto-immune encephalomyelitis. This finding demonstrates that microarray analysis provides leads to gene targets for MS that can be tested in animal models.

Animal Models

MS is similar to an autoimmune disease in mice called experimental autoimmune encephalomyelitis (EAE). In EAE, injection of myelin proteins triggers an immune response and generates an MS-like condition characterized by inflammation and demyelination. EAE is used as a model for studying the mechanisms of demyelination in mammals.

Researchers use genetically engineered mice to investigate the role of putative MS-linked genes. Izikson and co-workers at Harvard Medical School demonstrated that a cytokine receptor known as CCR2 plays a role in EAE. CCR2 helps recruit macrophages to sites of inflammation, and deletion of the gene for CCR2 completely cured EAE in experimental mice. Collaborators at the University of Copenhagen, Denmark; Cleveland Clinic Foundation, Cleveland, Ohio; and the University of California Los Angeles Medical Center are now investigating the role of CCR2 in people with MS.

Experimental mice can also yield valuable insight into the mechanisms of MS pathogenesis. Two of the original disease-modifying drugs, Avonex and Betaseron, are interferons whose mechanisms of action are still unknown. Teige and co-workers at the University of Lund, Sweden, showed that deletion of the gene for interferon-beta increased the severity of EAE in mice. They found that a lack of interferon-beta caused prolonged activation of microglia, resulting in chronic inflammation. This finding provided a critical starting point for investigators who study the role of interferon-beta in human cells.

The mouse model of MS has also been used to see if nature can provide new and better MS treatments. John Bright and co-workers at Vanderbilt University found that the production and activity of a proinflammatory cytokine, interleukin-12, is blocked by curcumin, a compound isolated from the plant *Curcuma longa*. In another study quercetin, a flavonoid that occurs naturally in many edible plants, also blocked the production of interleukin-12 by microglia, resulting in the reversal of symptoms associated with EAE. These results demonstrate that certain naturally occurring compounds are potent inhibitors of autoimmune inflammation and argue for the testing of these compounds in clinical trials.

Stem Cell Transplants

One of the most exciting new research areas is stem cell transplantation for the restoration of neurological function. Stem cells are present in the developing human embryo and at this stage are pluripotent—capable of differentiating into any cell type in the body. During natural development, stem cells are prompted to differentiate by the turning on of specific genes and the turning off of others. Researchers hope to be able to duplicate this process in adults, using stem cells to produce specific cell types that will replace damaged cells in the CNS.

Adults have multipotent stem cells, which are limited in their capacity to differentiate. Multipotent stem cells are present in tissues with high cellular turnover, such as the skin, the gut, and the bone marrow. Only recently have scientists been able to demonstrate the presence of multipotent stem cells in the adult brain. Stem cell progenitors of oligodendrocytes are, in fact, responsible for the limited remyelination that occurs after an MS exacerbation. Previously, it was thought that each tissue could only be regenerated from its own multipotent stem cell population. However, research during the last decade has shown that stem cells from blood and bone marrow can, under the right conditions, differentiate into many different cell types, including neurons and oligodendrocytes.

During the past decade, several clinical trials have reported mixed results for the effects of stem cells on MS. In these trials, researchers used stem cells derived from blood or bone marrow to replace the patients' immune systems. Injection of autologous stem cells following immunoablation generated a new repertoire of immune cells, and the effects on inflammatory demyelination were monitored. In most cases, the progression of MS was arrested and disability levels improved or remained stable. The number and size of brain lesions detected by MRI often decreased; at the very least, no new lesions were observed during the follow-up period (usually twelve to fifteen months). However, a number of treatment-related fatalities brought into question the benefits of stem cell therapy relative to its risks.

In the largest clinical trial conducted to date, the European Group for Blood and Marrow Transplantation reported on eighty-five MS patients who received autologous blood-derived stem cell transplants. Seven patients died, five from treatment-related complications and two from MS-related neurodegeneration. The results for surviving patients were promising: 21 percent showed improvement in their disability rating, and 74 percent were still progression-free after three years. In this and other trials, people with early stage relapsing-remitting MS or secondary progressive MS exhibited more improvement than people with primary progressive MS or very advanced neurodegeneration, most likely because this type of stem cell therapy specifically targets the inflammatory process that plays a role in the early stages of MS.

Once the survival rate improves, stem cell therapy for MS will likely become a common treatment. Stem cells are an obvious choice for supplementing remyelination after an exacerbation or for replacing damaged neurons. Since sites of damage are widespread throughout the CNS, and their locations differ between patients, it is hoped that intravenous delivery of autologous stem cells will result in migration of the cells to the proper locations. Preliminary evidence obtained by Eva Mezey and co-workers at the National Institutes of Health suggests that this is indeed what will happen. They examined postmortem brain samples of women who had received bone marrow transplants from men and found that Y-chromosome-containing cells had migrated into the brain and begun to differentiate.

Multipotent stem cells hold promise as a therapy for MS and other neurological diseases. They are less likely than pluripotent cells to lead to cancer via uncontrolled proliferation. Also, multipotent stem cells can be isolated from an individual and reinjected into that individual without causing an immune reaction, since they display only surface markers to which that person's immune system is already tolerant.

While extraction of stem cells from blood or bone marrow circumvents the need for brain surgery to get neural precursor cells, stem cell therapy presents some daunting challenges. The decision of which patients will benefit from this treatment is still a subject of debate. Secondary progressive MS, characterized more by neurodegeneration than inflammation, may not respond to stem cell treatment aimed at replacing a self-reactive immune system. Of concern to all MS patients is that the use of autologous stem cells may not circumvent the original problem of autoimmunity: that self-derived material is triggering an immune response. In autoimmune diseases, then, exogenous stem cells may be more effective, though suppression of the immune system would still be required to avoid rejection of the transplant. Additional challenges presented by stem cell therapy include purification of homogeneous stem cells from the isolated tissue and whether or not to attempt differentiation of pluripotent cells in the laboratory before reinjection into patients.

Stem cells seem very promising, but concerns remain with regard to this new technology. Among them are the potential of stem cell transplants to multiply unchecked and become malignant tumors; the possibility that introduction of new neurons into the CNS will overstimulate the system and trigger epileptic seizures; and the chance that autologous cells may express the same genes that predisposed the patient to MS in the first place. Researchers will have to proceed with caution while elucidating successful transplantation strategies.

The research outlook for MS is tremendously positive. The strategies described here will be integrated by scientists from around the world to produce new drugs and therapies for testing in clinical trials. A possible scenario: Microarray technology is used to identify genes of interest that are expressed in MS plaques. The results are published, and an independent research group chooses several different genes to test in transgenic mice. They determine that one of those genes encodes a protein that increases the severity of EAE in mice. Their collaborators are called upon to elucidate the structure of the protein and to design small molecule inhibitors of the protein. One small molecule has a protective effect against EAE when administered to mice. A pharmaceutical company then performs clinical trials to determine the effectiveness of the molecule in treating MS patients, and you read about the results in your monthly MS newsletter.

Appendix A

Internet Resources

www.nmss.org
The website of the National Multiple Sclerosis Society containing extensive information about MS, including treatment options, current research, and local MS chapters.

www.nlm.nih.gov/medlineplus/multiplesclerosis.html
A compilation of the latest news stories, overviews, research, and more on MS from MedlinePlus, the National Library of Medicine's consumer health site.

www.msfacts.org
The website of the Multiple Sclerosis Foundation, Inc., a service-based nonprofit organization whose mission is to ensure the best quality of life for those coping with MS.

www.mscare.org
The website of the Consortium of Multiple Sclerosis Centers, a multidisciplinary organization providing networking for health-care professionals specializing in the care of MS. CMSC also provides medical information for MS patients.

www.msaa.com
The website of the Multiple Sclerosis Association of America, a national and international nonprofit charitable organization serving those and the families of those with multiple sclerosis and other neurological diseases.

**www.ninds.nih.gov/disorders/multiple_sclerosis/
multiple_sclerosis.htm**
Information page on MS from the National Institute of
Neurological Disorders and Stroke.

medstat.med.utah.edu/kw/ms
An information site designed as an introduction to multiple sclerosis for medical students and physicians in training.

www.mult-sclerosis.org
A general information site compiled and maintained by
Paul Jones, a British MS patient. The site contains basic information on MS, including disease types, symptoms, diagnosis,
and treatments, and also highlights the personal experiences
of several MS patients.

Appendix B

Organizations

International Multiple Sclerosis Support Foundation
9136 E. Valencia Road
Suite 110, PMB 83
Tucson, AZ 85747
jsumption@imssf.org
www.jsumption.com/imssf/
Fax: 520-579-9473

Multiple Sclerosis Association of America
706 Haddonfield Road
Cherry Hill, NJ 08002
msaa@msaa.com
Tel: 856-488-4500/800-532-7667
Fax: 856-661-9797

Multiple Sclerosis Foundation
6350 North Andrews Avenue
Ft. Lauderdale, FL 33309-2130
support@msfocus.org
Tel: 954-776-6805/888-MSFOCUS (888-673-6287)
Fax: 954-351-0630

National Multiple Sclerosis Society
733 Third Avenue
6th Floor
New York, NY 10017-3288
nat@nmss.org
www.nationalmssociety.org

Tel: 212-986-3240/800-344-4867 (800-FIGHTMS)
Fax: 212-986-7981

American Autoimmune Related Diseases Association
22100 Gratiot Avenue
Eastpointe
East Detroit, MI 48201-2227
aarda@aol.com
www.aarda.org
Tel: 586-776-3900/800-598-4668
Fax: 586-776-3903

Well Spouse Foundation
63 West Main Street Suite H
Freehold, NJ 07728
info@wellspouse.org
www.wellspouse.org
Tel: 800-838-0879/732-577-8899
Fax: 732-577-8644

Accelerated Cure Project for Multiple Sclerosis/Boston Cure
Project for MS
300 Fifth Avenue
Waltham, MA 02451
info@bostoncure.org
www.bostoncure.org
Tel: 781-487-0008
Fax: 781-788-8118

Appendix C

MS Treatment Centers

Alabama
University of Alabama—Birmingham
619 19th Street
Department of Neurology
Birmingham, AL 35249
Telephone: 205-934-2402
Fax: 205-975-6030
www.neuro.uab.edu

Veterans Administration Medical Center—Birmingham
700 South 19th Street
Birmingham, AL 35233
Telephone: 205-933-8101

Veterans Administration Medical Center—Central Alabama
2400 Hospital Road
Tuskegee, AL 36083
Telephone: 334-727-0550, ext. 3
Fax: 334-724-6857

Veterans Administration Medical Center—Tuscaloosa
3701 Loop Road East
Tuscaloosa, AL 35404
Telephone: 205-554-2000

Arizona
Barrow Neurological Clinics
350 West Thomas Road 8BNI

Phoenix, AZ 85013
Telephone: 602-406-3390
Fax: 602-406-7161
www.thebarrow.com

Veterans Administration Medical Center—Phoenix—Carl
T. Hayden
650 E. Indian School Road
Phoenix, AZ 85012
Telephone: 602-222-6401
Fax: 602-200-6021

Veterans Administration Medical Center—Prescott
500 N. Highway 89 PM&R Service (117)
Prescott, AZ 86313
Telephone: 520-776-6087
Fax: 520-776-6172

Arkansas
Veterans Administration Medical Center—Little Rock
4300 West 7th Street
Little Rock, AR 72205
Telephone: 501-660-2070
Fax: 501-671-2514

California
East Bay Region Associates in Neurology MS Center
(EBRAIN MS Center)
3000 Colby Street, Suite 101, 201
Berkeley, CA 94705
Telephone: 510-849-0499
Fax: 510-849-0159

UCSF MS Center
350 Parnassus Avenue, Suite 908
San Francisco, CA 94117
Telephone: 415-514-1684
Fax: 415-514-2443

USC MS Comprehensive Care Center
1510 San Pablo Street, Room 637
Los Angeles, CA 90033
Telephone: 323-442-6870
Fax: 323-442-5773

Veterans Administration Medical Center—West LA MS
Treatment Program
11301 Wilshire Boulevard
Neurology W127
Los Angeles, CA 90073
Telephone: 310-268-3013
Fax: 310-268-4611

Veterans Administration Medical Center—Sepulveda
16111 Plummer Street
Sepulveda, CA 91343
Telephone: 818-895-9473
Fax: 818-895-5801

Veterans Administration Medical Center—Fresno
2615 East Clinton Avenue
Neurology 127
Fresno, CA 93703
Telephone: 209-228-5328
Fax: 209-228-6943

Veterans Administration Medical Center—Palo Alto
3801 Miranda Avenue
Palo Alto, CA 94304
Telephone: 650-493-5000
Fax: 650-852-3280

Colorado
Colorado Springs Neurological Association, PC
415 W. Rockrimmon Boulevard, Suite 400
Colorado Springs, CO 80919
Telephone: 719-598-9991
Fax: 719-598-2044

Rocky Mountain MS Center
701 East Hampden Avenue, #530
Englewood, CO 80113
Telephone: 303-788-7667
Fax: 303-788-8854
www.mscenter.org

The Heuga Center
27 Main Street, Suite 303
Edwards, CO 81632
Telephone: 970-926-1290
Fax: 970-926-1295
www.heuga.org

University of Colorado Multiple Sclerosis Center
4200 East Ninth Avenue, Box B183
Denver, CO 80262
Telephone: 303-315-8760
Fax: 303-315-5867

Veterans Administration Medical Center—Denver
1055 Clermont Street
PMRS 117
Denver, CO 80220
Telephone: 303-393-2819
Fax: 303-393-5164

Connecticut

Veterans Administration Medical Center—Connecticut
Healthcare System
950 Campbell Avenue, Firm B2
West Haven, CT 06516
Telephone: 203-932-5711 ext. 2268
Fax: 203-937-4918

Yale University School of Medicine MS Clinic
40 Temple Street, Suite 7-I
New Haven, CT 06510
Telephone: 203-764-4294
Fax: 203-764-4288

Delaware

Veterans Administration Medical Center—Wilmington
1601 Kirkwood Highway
Wilmington, DE 19805
Telephone: 302-994-2511
Fax: 302-633-5582

District of Columbia

Georgetown University MS Center
3800 Reservoir Road NW, One Bles—Department of
Neurology
Washington, DC 20007

Telephone: 202-784-1762
Fax: 202-784-2261
www.mscenter.georgetown.edu

Veterans Administration Medical Center—Washington, DC
50 Irving Street, NW, 3B West
Washington, DC 20422
Telephone: 202-745-8148
Fax: 202-745-8231

Florida
Doctors Hospital MS Center
5000 University Drive
Coral Gables, FL 33146
Telephone: 305-728-4358
Fax: 305-595-6638

MS Comprehensive Care Center of Central Florida
6001 Vineland Road, Suite 116
Orlando, FL 32819
Telephone: 407-352-5434
Fax: 407-345-9765
www.mscentralfl.com

University of Miami Multiple Sclerosis Center
1501 NW 9th Avenue
NPF Building, 2nd Floor
Miami, FL 33136
Telephone: 305-243-1088
Fax: 305-243-1119

Veterans Administration Medical Center—Miami
1201 NW 16th Street

Miami, FL 33125
Telephone: 305-324-3151
Fax: 305-324-3210

Veterans Administration Medical Center—Tampa
13000 Bruce B. Downs Boulevard
Tampa, FL 33612
Telephone: 813-972-7517
Fax: 813-978-5913

Georgia
Medical College of Georgia
1120 15th Street, BB-3516
Augusta, GA 30912
Telephone: 706-721-1886
Fax: 706-721-1962
www.neuro.mcg.edu

MS Center at Shepherd
2020 Peachtree Road NW
Atlanta, GA 30309
Telephone: 404-350-7392
Fax: 404-350-7526

Illinois
Loyola University of Chicago MS Clinic
2160 South First Avenue
Maywood, IL 60153
Telephone: 708-216-3772
Fax: 708-216-5617

Rush Multiple Sclerosis Center
1725 West Harrison Street, Suite 309

Chicago, IL 60612
Telephone: 312-942-8011
Fax: 312-942-2253
www.rush.edu/rumc/page-1099611537766.html

University of Chicago MS Clinic
5841 S. Maryland Avenue, MC2030
Chicago, IL 60637
Telephone: 773-702-6386
Fax: 773-702-9060

Veterans Administration Medical Center—Chicago Lakeside
333 East Huron Street
Chicago, IL 60611
Telephone: 312-943-6600 ext. 40
Fax: 312-640-2153

Veterans Administration Medical Center—Chicago Westside
820 S. Damen Avenue
Department of Physical Medicine
Chicago, IL 60612
Telephone: 312-666-6500
Fax: 312-455-5821

Veterans Administration Medical Center—Hines
PO Box 5000
Department of Neurology 127
Hines, IL 60141
Telephone: 708-202-8387 ext. 22
Fax: 708-202-7936

Veterans Administration Medical Center—North Chicago
3001 Greenbay Road

North Chicago, IL 60064
Telephone: 847-688-1900 ext. 8
Fax: 847-578-3863

Indiana
Fort Wayne Neurological Center
2622 Lake Avenue
MS Center of Northeast Indiana
Fort Wayne, IN 46805
Telephone: 219-460-3100
Fax: 219-460-3130
www.fwnc.com

Indiana Center for MS & Neuroimmunopathologic
Disorders
8424 Naab Road, Suite 1A
Indianapolis, IN 46260
Telephone: 317-614-3100
Fax: 317-614-3111
www.icmsnd.com

Indiana University Multiple Sclerosis Center
541 Clinical Drive, CL292
Indianapolis, IN 46202
Telephone: 317-274-4030
Fax: 317-274-3619

Veterans Administration Medical Center—Indianapolis
1481 West 10th Street
VAMC Neurology Service (127)
Indianapolis, IN 46202
Telephone: 317-554-0227
Fax: 317-554-0215

Iowa
Ruan MS Center
1111 6th Avenue, Suite W4
Des Moines, IA 50314
Telephone: 515-643-4500
Fax: 515-643-4505

Kansas
University of Kansas MS Center
1033B Wescoe KU Hospital
3901 Rainbow Boulevard
Kansas City, KS 66160
Telephone: 913-588-6970
Fax: 913-588-6965

Veterans Administration Medical Center—Topeka
2200 Gage Boulevard
Topeka, KS 66622
Telephone: 785-350-3111
Fax: 785-350-4429

Kentucky
Baptist Hospital East MS Center
4002 Kresge Way
Louisville, KY 40207
Telephone: 502-896-7695
Fax: 502-896-7469

Louisville Comprehensive Care MS Center
250 East Liberty Street, Suite 202
Louisville, KY 40202
Telephone: 502-589-6172
Fax: 502-589-0544

Louisiana
LSU Multiple Sclerosis Clinic
1542 Tulane Avenue
Room 220, Department of Neurology
New Orleans, LA 70112
Telephone: 504-568-4082
Fax: 504-568-4084

Our Lady of Lourdes MS Center
611 St. Landry Street
Lafayette, LA 70506
Telephone: 337-289-4978
Fax: 337-289-2883

Veterans Administration Medical Center—Alexandria
PO Box 69004 Medical Svc (III)
Alexandria, LA 71301
Telephone: 318-473-0010 ext. 2646
Fax: 318-483-0065

Veterans Administration Medical Center—New Orleans
Neurology Section HF165
1601 Perdido Street
New Orleans, LA 70146
Telephone: 504-589-5227
Fax: 504-589-5232

Maine
Multiple Sclerosis Center of Maine
49 Spring Street
Scarborough, ME 04074
Telephone: 207-883-1414
Fax: 207-883-1010
www.maineneurology.neurohub.net

Veterans Administration Medical Center—Togus
240 River Road
Bowdoinham, ME 04008
Telephone: 207-623-8411 ext. 5501
Fax: 207-621-4819

Maryland
Maryland Center for Multiple Sclerosis
11 S. Paca Street, 4th Floor
Baltimore, MD 21201
Telephone: 410-328-7601
Fax: 410-328-5425

VA MS Center of Excellence—East
(Veterans Administration Medical Center—Baltimore)
Neurology Service 127
10 North Greene Street
Baltimore, MD 21201
Telephone: 410-605-7480
Fax: 410-605-7937
www.va.gov/ms

Massachusetts
Brigham and Women's Hospital
77 Avenue Louis Pasteur, HIM 730
Boston, MA 02115
Telephone: 617-525-5300
Fax: 617-525-5252

Mount Auburn Hospital MS Care Center
330 Mount Auburn Street
Cambridge, MA 02238
Telephone: 617-499-5014
Fax: 617-499-5441

Newton Wellesley MS Center
2014 Washington Street
Newton, MA 02162
Telephone: 617-969-1723
Fax: 617-630-0860

Sturdy Memorial Hospital MS Center
P.O. Box 2963
211 Park Street
Attleboro, MA 02703
Telephone: 508-236-7170
Fax: 508-236-7610
www.sturdymemorial.org

Veterans Administration Medical Center—West Roxbury
221 Longwood Avenue, LMRC 1024
West Roxbury, MA 02132
Telephone: 617-323-7700 ext. 68

Michigan
Michigan Institute for Neurological Disorders
28595 Orchard Lake Road, Suite 200
Farmington Hills, MI 48334
Telephone: 248-553-0010
Fax: 248-553-5957
www.mindonline.com

MS Clinical and Research at Wayne State University
4201 St. Antoine, Suite 8D
Department of Neurology
Detroit, MI 48201
Telephone: 313-577-1249
Fax: 313-745-4216

Minnesota
MS Treatment and Research Center
4225 Golden Valley Road
Golden Valley, MN 55422
Telephone: 763-588-0661
Fax: 763-287-2310

Schapiro Center for MS at the Minneapolis Clinic of
Neurology
4225 Golden Valley Road
Golden Valley, MN 55422
Telephone: 763-588-0661
Fax: 612-672-6504

St. Mary's/Duluth Clinic—Comprehensive MS Center
400 E. 3rd Street Neurology
Duluth, MN 55805
Telephone: 218-786-3925
Fax: 218-722-4302

Veterans Administration Medical Center—Minneapolis
One Veterans Drive
Minneapolis, MN 55417
Telephone: 612-725-2047
Fax: 612-725-2068

Mississippi
University of Mississippi Medical Center
2500 N. State Street
Neurology L207
Jackson, MS 39216
Telephone: 601-984-5500
Fax: 601-984-5503

Missouri
The John L. Trotter Multiple Sclerosis Center
660 South Euclid Avenue, Campus Box 8111
St. Louis, MO 63110
Telephone: 314-362-3293
Fax: 314-747-1345

Montana
Northern Rockies Multiple Sclerosis Center
2900 12th Avenue N., Suite 401-E
Billings, MT 59101
Telephone: 406-237-4280
Fax: 406-237-4291
www.svh-mt.org/our_health_services/neurology_
ms_clinic.asp

Nebraska
UNMC MS Center
982045 Nebraska Medical Center
Omaha, NE
Telephone: 402-559-7857
Fax: 402-559-3545

Nevada
Washoe Institute for Neurosciences MS Center
77 Pringle Way, CC-3
Reno, NV 89502
Telephone: 775-982-4602
Fax: 775-324-6015

New Hampshire
Veterans Administration Medical Center—Manchester
718 Smyth Road
Spinal Cord Injury and Disorders #122

Manchester, NH 03104
Telephone: 603-624-4366 ext. 6320

MS Clinic of the Upper Valley
106 Hanover Street
Lebanon, NH 03766
Telephone: 603-448-0447
Fax: 603-448-1089

New Jersey
Kessler Medical Rehabilitation Research and Education
Corporation
1199 Pleasant Valley Way
West Orange, NJ 07052
Telephone: 973-243-6974
Fax: 973-243-6984

MS Center at Centrastate Medical Center
901 West Main Street
Freehold, NJ 07728
Telephone: 732-294-2505
Fax: 732-761-8084
www.centrastate.com/body.cfm?id=988

Veterans Administration Medical Center—East Orange
185 S. Orange Avenue, MSB-H506
East Orange, NJ 07018
Telephone: 973-676-1000 ext. 14
Fax: 973-676-1648

Gimbel MS Center
718 Teaneck Road
Teaneck, NJ 07666
www.msccc.org

New Mexico
MS Specialty Clinic of New Mexico
The MIND Imaging Center
1201 Yale Boulevard, NE
Albuquerque, NM 87131
Telephone: 505-272-0760
Fax: 505-272-1816

Veterans Administration Medical Center—Albuquerque
1501 San Pedro Drive SW
Albuquerque, NM 87108
Telephone: 505-256-2752
Fax: 505-256-2870

New York
Alpha Neurology
27 New Dorp Lane
Staten Island, NY 10306
Telephone: 718-667-3800
Fax: 718-667-3590

Capital Neurological Associates
650 Warren Street
Albany, NY 12208
Telephone: 518-459-8106
Fax: 518-489-6441
www.capitalneuro.com

Center For Multiple Sclerosis at Albany Medical College
47 New Scotland Avenue, Neurology MC-70
Albany, NY 12208
Telephone: 518-262-5226
Fax: 518-262-6261
www.amc.edu/neurosciences/index.htm

Corinne Goldsmith Dickinson Center for MS
5 East 98th Street, Box 1138
New York, NY 10029
Telephone: 212-241-6854
Fax: 212-423-0440

Hospital for Joint Diseases at NYU
301 E. 17th Street, Room #1615 NE
New York, NY 10003
Telephone: 212-598-6305
Fax: 212-598-6214

Jacobs Neurological Institute/Baird MS Research Center
100 High Street
Buffalo, NY 14203
Telephone: 716-859-7540
Fax: 716-859-2430

Maimonides Multiple Sclerosis Care Center
4802 Tenth Avenue, Neurology
Brooklyn, NY 11219
Telephone: 718-283-7470
Fax: 718-283-8836

MS Care Center at Center Health Care
314 South Manning Boulevard
Albany, NY 12208
Telephone: 518-437-5963
Fax: 518-437-5963

Rochester Multiple Sclerosis Center
601 Elmwood Avenue, Box 605
Rochester, NY 14642

Telephone: 585-275-0833
Fax: 585-273-2857

Stony Brook MS Comprehensive Care Center
HSC T12-020, Department of Neurology
Stony Brook, NY 11794
Telephone: 631-444-8188
Fax: 631-444-1474

SUNY Upstate Medical University
750 E. Adams Street, Department of Neurology
Syracuse, NY 13210
Telephone: 315-464-5356
Fax: 315-464-5355

Veterans Administration Medical Center—Buffalo
3495 Bailey Avenue
Buffalo, NY 14215
Telephone: 716-862-3653
Fax: 716-862-3475

Veterans Administration Medical Center—New York
423 East 23rd Street
New York, NY 10010
Telephone: 212-951-3320
Fax: 212-951-3246

Veterans Administration Medical Center—Albany
113 Holland Avenue, Mail Code 111G
Albany, NY 12208
Telephone: 518-626-6497
Fax: 518-626-6495

Veterans Administration Medical Center—Brooklyn
800 Poly Place
Brooklyn, NY 11209
Telephone: 718-630-3724
Fax: 718-439-3577

Veterans Administration Medical Center—Northport
79 Middleville Road
Northport, NY 11768
Telephone: 631-754-7962

North Carolina
CMC Myers Park Clinic—MS Center
1350 South Kings Drive
Charlotte, NC 28207
Telephone: 704-446-1900
Fax: 704-446-1289

Triangle Multiple Sclerosis Center
1540 Sunday Drive
Raleigh, NC 27607
Telephone: 919-782-3456
Fax: 919-420-1688

Veterans Administration Medical Center—Durham
508 Fulton Street, Mail Code 117
Durham, NC 27705
Telephone: 919-286-6874
Fax: 919-416-5913

Wake Forest University MS Center
Medical Center Boulevard
P.O. Box 1078

Winston-Salem, NC 27157
Telephone: 336-713-8611
Fax: 336-713-8588

North Dakota
Altru Health Institute
1300 South Columbia Road
P.O. Box 6002
Grand Forks, ND 58206
Telephone: 701-780-2466
Fax: 701-780-2599

MeritCare NeuroScience
700 1st Avenue South
Fargo, ND 58103
Telephone: 701-234-4036
Fax: 701-234-4151

Ohio
Mellen Center for MS Treatment & Research
9500 Euclid Avenue, U-10
Cleveland, OH 44195
Telephone: 216-444-6800
Fax: 216-445-7013

Ohio State University MS Center
1654 Upham Drive, 449 Means Hall
Columbus, OH 43210
Telephone: 614-293-4964
Fax: 614-293-6111

Riverhills Multiple Sclerosis Center
111 Wellington Place
Cincinnati, OH 45219

Telephone: 513-487-4878
Fax: 513-241-6053

Veterans Administration Medical Center—Cleveland
10701 East Boulevard
Cleveland, OH 44106
Telephone: 216-421-3040
Fax: 216-421-3040

Veterans Administration Medical Center—Dayton
4100 West Third Street
Dayton, OH 45428
Telephone: 513-262-2161
Fax: 513-267-3983

Veterans Administration Medical Center—Ohio
17273 State Route 104 PM & R 117
Chillicothe, OH 45601
Telephone: 740-773-1141 ext. 7638
Fax: 740-772-7144

Waddell MS Center—University of Cincinnati
222 Piedmont Avenue, Suite 3200
Cincinnati, OH 45219
Telephone: 513-475-8730
Fax: 513-475-0833

Oklahoma
Veterans Administration Medical Center—Oklahoma City
921 NE 13th Street, Neurosciences Center
Oklahoma City, OK 73104
Telephone: 405-270-0501 ext. 3896
Fax: 405-271-5723

Oregon
Oregon Health and Science University
MS Center of Oregon
3181 SW Sam Jackson Park Road
Portland, OR 97239
Telephone: 503-494-7321
Fax: 503-494-7242

Veterans Administration Medical Center—Portland
3710 SW US Veterans Hospital Road (153)
PO Box 1034
Portland, OR 97207
Telephone: 503-220-8262 ext. 57260
Fax: 503-220-3439

Pennsylvania
Allegheny MS Treatment Center
420 East North Avenue, Suite 206
Pittsburgh, PA 15212
Telephone: 412-321-2162
Fax: 412-321-5073

Geisinger Medical Center MS Clinic
100 N. Academy Street
Danville, PA 17822
Telephone: 570-271-6694
Fax: 570-271-5874

Health South Rehab Hospital of Erie
143 East 2nd Street
Erie, PA 16507

Good Shepherd Rehabilitation MS
820 South Fifth Street

Wellness Program and MS Day Hospital
Allentown, PA 18103
Telephone: 610-776-3315
Fax: 610-776-3168

MS Center of the Lehigh Valley at Lehigh Valley Hospital
1210 S. Cedar Crest Boulevard, Suite 1200
Allentown, PA 18103
Telephone: 610-402-8420
Fax: 610-402-1689
www.lvhhn.org/services/excellence/ms_center/

Multiple Sclerosis Institute
1740 South Street, Suite 401
Philadelphia, PA 19146
Telephone: 215-985-2245
Fax: 215-985-2250

Thomas Jefferson University Comprehensive MS Center
1025 Walnut Street, Suite 310
Philadelphia, PA 19107
Telephone: 215-955-7310
Fax: 215-503-2990

UPHS Comprehensive MS Center
3400 Spruce Street, Department of Neurology
Philadelphia, PA 19104
Telephone: 215-349-8110
Fax: 215-349-5579

University of Pittsburgh MS Center
3471 Fifth Avenue, Suite 810
Pittsburgh, PA 15213

Telephone: 412-692-4914
Fax: 412-692-4897

Veterans Administration Medical Center—Lebanon
1700 S. Lincoln Avenue
Lebanon, PA 17042
Telephone: 717-272-6621 [pager]
Fax: 717-228-5982

Veterans Administration Medical Center—Philadelphia
University & Woodland Avenues
Philadelphia, PA 19104
Telephone: 215-823-5850
Fax: 215-823-5969

Veterans Administration Medical Center—Pittsburgh
University Drive C
Pittsburgh, PA 15240
Telephone: 412-688-6185
Fax: 412-688-6920

South Carolina
Carolina Neurology
541 Floyd Road
Spartanburg, SC 29307
Telephone: 864-585-6179
Fax: 864-583-5403

Medical University of SC MS Center
Veterans Administration Medical Center—Charleston
96 Jonathan Lucas Street, Suite 309
Charleston, SC 29401
Telephone: 843-792-3221
Fax: 843-792-8626

Veterans Administration Medical Center—WJB Dorn
6439 Garners Ferry Road
Columbia, SC 29209
Telephone: 803-776-4000 ext. 62
Fax: 803-695-7932

Tennessee
St. Thomas Multiple Sclerosis Center
4230 Harding Road, Suite 807
Nashville, TN 37205
Telephone: 615-467-6256
Fax: 615-467-6258

Texas
The Institute of Rehabilitation and Research (TIRR)
1333 Moursund Street
Houston, TX 77030
Telephone: 713-797-7561
Fax: 713-797-7564
www.tirr.org

The Maxine Mesinger MS Clinic
6501 Fannin Street, Suite NB100
Houston, TX 77030
Telephone: 713-798-7707
Fax: 713-798-6273
www.bcm.tmc.edu/neurol

VA North Texas Healthcare System
4500 S. Lancaster Road
Dallas, TX 75216
Telephone: 214-857-0114
Fax: 214-857-1759

UT Southwestern Medical Center of Dallas
5323 Harry Hines Boulevard
Dallas, TX 75390
Telephone: 214-648-9030
Fax: 214-648-9129

Veterans Administration Medical Center/University of Texas
Health Science Center
7703 Floyd Curl Drive
San Antonio, TX 78284
Telephone: 210-617-5161
Fax: 210-567-4659

Utah
Veterans Administration Medical Center—Salt Lake City
500 Foothill Drive
Salt Lake City, UT 84148
Telephone: 801-584-1292
Fax: 801-582-6908

Western Neurological Associates
1151 East 3900 South
Salt Lake City, UT 84124
Telephone: 801-262-3441
Fax: 801-269-9005

Vermont
Neurological Research Center, Inc.
140 Hospital Drive, Suite 210
Bennington, VT 05201
Telephone: 800-447-7577
Fax: 802-447-2676

Northern New England Multiple Sclerosis Center
1 South Prospect Street, 6th Floor UHC
Burlington, VT 05401
Telephone: 802-847-4589
Fax: 802-847-9489

Virginia
James Q. Miller Consultative MS Clinic
Fontaine Adult Neurology Clinic
P.O. Box 801018
Charlottesville, VA
Telephone: 804-243-5931
Fax: 804-982-3544

Neurology Center of Fairfax
3020 Hamaker Court, Suite 400
Fairfax, VA 22031
Telephone: 703-876-0811
Fax: 703-876-0832

Northern Virginia Neurologic Associates, Ltd.
1635 N. George Mason Drive, Suite 420
Arlington, VA 22205
Telephone: 703-536-4000
Fax: 703-527-4339

Veterans Administration Medical Center—Salem
1970 Roanoke Boulevard
Salem, VA 24153
Telephone: 540-982-2463
Fax: 540-224-1963

Washington
Holy Family Hospital MS Center
5901 N. Lidgerwood Street, Suite B-25
Spokane, WA 99207
Telephone: 509-489-5019
Fax: 509-489-1812

MSHub Medical Group
1100 Olive Way
Seattle, WA 98101
Telephone: 206-262-0110
Fax: 206-262-0303

Overlake Hospital MS Center
1035 116th Avenue, NE
Bellevue, WA 98004
Telephone: 425-688-5070
Fax: 425-688-5657

University of Washington
Box 356490, Rehabilitation Medicine
Seattle, WA 98195
Telephone: 206-543-7272
Fax: 206-685-3244

Veterans Administration Medical Center—Seattle
1145 22nd Avenue E
Seattle, WA 98112
Telephone: 206-277-3452
Fax: 206-764-2263

Virginia Mason Multiple Sclerosis Center
1100 9th Avenue, Box 900 MS:X7 NEU

Seattle, WA 98101
Telephone: 206-223-6753
Fax: 206-625-7240

Wisconsin
Marshfield MS Center
1000 North Oak Avenue
Marshfield, WI 54449
Telephone: 715-387-5351
Fax: 715-387-5727

Medical College of Wisconsin
9200 West Wisconsin Avenue, Neurology
Milwaukee, WI 53226
Telephone: 414-805-5203
Fax: 414-259-0469
www.mcw.edu/display/router.asp?DocID=1997

Canada
Dalhousie University MS Research Unit
5790 University Avenue, Room 114, DMSRU
Halifax, NS, CA
Telephone: 902-422-7817

G. F. Strong Rehab Center
4255 Laurel Street
Vancouver, BC, CA
Telephone: 604-734-1313 ext. 24
Fax: 604-737-6359

Hamilton MS Clinic
1200 Main Street W., Room 4 U3
Hamilton, ON, CA

Telephone: 905-521-2100 ext. 76
Fax: 905-521-2656

MS Center for the Greater Quebec Area
525 Boul Hamel I.R.D. P.Q.
Quebec, PQ, CA
Telephone: 418-529-9141
Fax: 418-649-3703

NF Multiple Sclerosis Clinic
300 Prince Philip Drive
St. John's, NF, CA
Telephone: 709-777-6594
Fax: 709-777-6656

Northern Health—Porch MS Clinic
1475 Edmonton Street
Prince George, BC, CA
Telephone: 250-565-2304
Fax: 250-565-2662

Ottawa Hospital MS Clinic
501 Smyth Road, Box 606
Ottawa, ON, CA
Telephone: 613-737-8532
Fax: 613-739-6631

UBC Multiple Sclerosis Clinic
S159-2211 Wesbrook Mall
Vancouver, BC, CA
Telephone: 604-822-7696
Fax: 604-822-0758

University of Calgary MS Clinic
1403 29 Street, NW
12th Floor, Room C1223

Foothills Medical Centre Building
Calgary, AB, CA
Telephone: 403-944-4241
Fax: 403-283-2270

Puerto Rico
Veterans Administration Medical Center—San Juan
10 Calle Casia, Neurology Section
San Juan 921, PR
Telephone: 787-641-7582 ext. 3
Fax: 787-641-4561

Glossary

Action potential   A cascade of ions into and out of an axon that produces a nerve impulse.

Adhesion molecule   Any of a family of proteins (cellular adhesion molecules [CAMs], integrins, and selectins) that mediate cell adhesion and migration across capillary walls into surrounding tissue.

Allele   Any of the alternative forms of a gene that occur at a given site.

Alternative medicine   Treatments used in place of conventional medicines. Various systems of healing or treating disease (such as homeopathy, chiropractic, naturopathy, Ayurveda, or faith healing) that are not included in the traditional curricula taught in medical schools of the U.S and Britain.

Amino acid   Chemical unit that, when linked with other amino acids in a linear chain, forms a protein.

Antibody   Any of a large number of proteins that are produced normally by specialized B cells after stimulation by an antigen and act specifically against the antigen in an immune response. They typically consist of four subunits including two heavy chains and two light chains-also called **immunoglobulin**.

Antigen   A substance capable of stimulating an immune response.

Antigen-presenting cells (APCs)   Phagocytes that break down antigens into their molecular components and present their epitopes to T cells.

Association neuron   A neuron that conducts nerve impulses within the central nervous system, connecting sensory and motor neurons.

Astrocyte   A star-shaped neuroglial cell that reinforces the blood-brain barrier.

Ataxia   The inability to coordinate voluntary muscular movements.

Autoimmunity   A condition in which the body produces an immune response against its own tissue constituents.

Autologous   Self-derived, as an autologous antigen.

Avonex   Brand name for interferon beta-1a. One of the disease-modifying MS therapies.

Axon   A long and single neuronal process that conducts impulses away from the cell body.

B cell   Any of the lymphocytes that have antibody molecules on the surface and become antibody-secreting cells when activated.

Betaseron   Brand name for interferon beta-1b. One of the disease-modifying MS therapies.

Blood-brain barrier (BBB)   A naturally occurring barrier created by the modification of brain capillaries by formation of tight cell-to-cell contacts. The BBB prevents many substances from leaving the blood and crossing the capillary walls into the brain tissues.

Central nervous system (CNS)   The part of the nervous system that consists of the brain and spinal cord, to which sensory impulses are transmitted and from which motor impulses pass out, and that supervises and coordinates the activity of the entire nervous system.

Cerebrospinal fluid (CSF)   A liquid that is secreted from the blood into the lateral ventricles of the brain and that serves chiefly to maintain uniform pressure within the brain and spinal cord.

Chromosome   Linear structure, made up of DNA and protein molecules, that houses the genes.

Complementary medicine   Any treatment regimen that supplements traditional prescription medicine.

Copaxone   Brand name for glatiramer acetate, or copolymer-1. A disease-modifying MS therapy consisting of random polymers of the amino acids glutamic acid, lysine, alanine, and tyrosine.

Cytokine   Any of a class of immunoregulatory proteins (such as interleukins, tumor necrosis factor, and interferons) that are secreted by cells of the immune system.

Demyelination   The state resulting from the loss or destruction of myelin, or the process of such loss or destruction.

Dendrites   The branched processes that conduct impulses toward the cell body of a neuron.

Disulfide bond   A covalent bond between two sulfur atoms that holds together, among other things, the heavy and light amino acid chains of an antibody.

DNA   Deoxyribonucleic acid. The chemical of which genes are made.

DNA microarray   A two-dimensional support to which DNA is linked and that is used to detect gene expression.

Dominant   An allele that produces its phenotype 100 percent of the time.

Endogenous   Produced or contained within.

Endothelial cell   The type of cell that covers a free surface or lines a tube or cavity (such as a blood vessel) and serves to enclose and protect.

Epidemiology   A branch of medical science that deals with the incidence, distribution, and control of disease in a population.

Epistasis   Suppression of phenotype by a nonallelic gene.

Epitope   A molecular region on the surface of an antigen capable of eliciting an immune response.

Epitope spreading   A theory of induction of autoimmunity in MS where chronic inflammation releases endogenous cell components that elicit an immune response from self-reactive T cells.

Estriol   The main estrogen secreted by the placenta during pregnancy.

Exacerbation   A period of time during which MS symptoms become more severe.

Exogenous   Produced or contained outside.

Experimental autoimmune encephalitis (EAE)   An inflammatory autoimmune disease that has been induced in laboratory animals, especially mice, by injecting them with diseased tissue from affected animals or with myelin basic protein. Because of the similarity of its pathology to MS in humans, it is used as an animal model in studying this condition.

Gadolinium   A magnetic metallic element of the rare-earth group, symbol *Gd.*

Gene   A sequence of nucleotide bases on a chromosome that encodes a single protein or RNA molecule. The physical and functional unit of heredity.

Genetic association study   A technique that determines whether or not a specific allele occurs more frequently in MS patients than in the general population.

Haplotype   A group of alleles on a single chromosome that are closely enough linked to be inherited as a unit.

Herb   A plant or plant part valued for its medicinal, savory, or aromatic qualities.

Human leukocyte antigen (HLA)   Any of various proteins that are encoded by genes of the major histocompatibility complex in humans and are found on the surface of many cell types (as white blood cells). A cell's HLA identifies it as "self" or "nonself" to the immune system.

Immigration effect   The change in MS risk that occurs when a population moves from a region of high incidence to one of low incidence, or vice versa.

Immunoglobulin   See **antibody**.

Incidence   The rate of occurrence of new cases of a particular disease in a population being studied.

Inflammation   A local response to cellular injury that is marked by increased blood flow, leukocyte infiltration, redness, heat, pain, swelling, and often loss of function and that serves as a mechanism initiating an immune response in damaged tissue.

Innervation   The distribution of nerves to or in a part of the body.

Interferons   One family of cytokines that is especially involved in viral resistance.

Interleukins   One family of cytokines that is produced and secreted by phagocytes and lymphocytes and that, among other things, mediates inflammation.

Leukocytes   White blood cells, including phagocytes, lymphocytes, and auxiliary cells.

Linkage   The proximity of genes on the same chromosome. The closer they are, the more likely they are to be inherited together.

Linkage analysis   A technique that uses linkage between genes to identify their association with a trait or condition.

Linkage disequilibrium   The state in which two genes are inherited together more often than expected based on the distance between them.

Lymphocytes   Cells that originate from bone marrow stem cells and differentiate in lymphoid tissue, primarily B cells and T cells.

Macrophage A phagocytic cell that may be fixed or freely motile and functions in the protection of the body against infection and noxious substances.

Magnetic resonance imaging (MRI) A noninvasive diagnostic technique that produces computerized images of internal body tissues and is based on nuclear magnetic resonance of atoms within the body induced by the application of radio waves.

McDonald criteria The newest diagnostic criteria for different types of MS.

Meiosis The process of cellular division that produces sperm or egg cells.

Microglia Neuroglia, consisting of small cells with few processes, that are scattered throughout the central nervous system and have a phagocytic function.

Mineral A naturally occurring, solid homogeneous crystalline chemical element or compound.

Mitoxantrone A small tricyclic anticancer agent that has immunosuppressant activity. See also **Novantrone**.

Molecular mimicry A theory of induction of autoimmunity in MS in which exogenous antigens mimic "self" structures, stimulating T cells to produce an immune response.

Monoparesis Paralysis affecting only one limb.

Mortality rate The number of deaths in a population in a given time or place. Usually expressed as deaths/100,000 persons/year.

Motor neuron A neuron that conducts nerve impulses from the central nervous system to the parts of the body capable of responding, such as muscles or glands.

MS attack An exacerbation of MS symptoms.

MS lesion A discoloration in the white matter of the brain indicative of demyelination.

MS plaque   A lesion in brain tissue that is characteristic of MS and indicative of demyelination.

Multipotent   Term used to describe a stem cell that has the ability to differentiate into any of several different cell types.

Myelin   A soft white fatty substance produced by oligodendrocytes that forms an insulating sheath around axons.

Natalizumab   A bioengineered monoclonal antibody used to inhibit cell adhesion during inflammation.

Nerve impulse   The electronic signal transmitted from the cell body of a neuron to its terminus. Also called an **action potential**.

Neuroglia   Any of the neuron-supporting cell types within the central nervous system.

Neuron   One of the cells that constitute nervous tissue and that have the property of transmitting and receiving nerve impulses.

Nodes of Ranvier   Interruptions in the myelin sheath that surrounds axons. Ion channels are located at the nodes of Ranvier, facilitating the conduction of nerve impulses.

Novantrone   Brand name of **mitoxantrone,** an anticancer drug used to suppress immune cells that attack the myelin sheath.

Oligodendrocyte   A neuroglial cell responsible for producing the myelin sheath.

Optic neuritis   Inflammation of the optic nerve.

Paraparesis   Partial paralysis affecting both lower limbs.

Penetrance   The proportion of individuals of a particular genotype that express its phenotype.

Peptide   A short (about 5–30 units) amino acid chain.

Perivascular foot   An extension of an astrocyte that surrounds a blood vessel.

Phagocyte   A leukocyte that engulfs and consumes foreign material (such as microorganisms) and cellular debris.

Phenotype   The detectable properties of an organism that are produced by the interaction of the genotype and the environment.

Placebo   An inert or innocuous substance used in controlled experiments testing the efficacy of another substance.

Pluripotent   Term used to describe a stem cell whose developmental fate is not yet fixed; it may differentiate into any of many different cell types.

Precursor   A chemical or cell that precedes another of its kind in developmental sequence.

Prevalence   The percentage of a population with a particular disease at a given time.

Primary progressive MS   A subtype of MS characterized by slow worsening of symptoms with no observable attacks.

Progressive relapsing MS   A subtype of MS characterized by slow worsening and acute attacks of increasing severity.

Rebif   Brand name of interferon beta-1a. Chemically identical to Avonex, it is used as a disease-modifying therapy for MS.

Recessive gene   A gene whose phenotype is not expressed unless two identical copies are present.

Relapsing-remitting MS   A subtype of MS characterized by distinct exacerbations separated by periods of full recovery.

RNA   Ribonucleic acid. The single-stranded nucleic acid intermediate in the synthesis of proteins from DNA.

Secondary progressive MS   A subtype of MS characterized by intermittent attacks and periods of recovery in which some disability is retained.

Sensory neuron   A neuron that conducts nerve impulses from the body via the five senses to the central nervous system.

Single nucleotide polymorphism (SNP), pronounced "snip"   A variant DNA sequence in which a single nucleotide has been replaced by another. SNPs may account for different disease susceptibilities in a population and can serve as genetic markers.

Spasticity   A condition characterized by strong muscular contraction with increased tendon reflexes.

Statins   Any of a group of drugs (e.g., simvastatin) that inhibit the synthesis of cholesterol and promote the production of low-density lipoprotein-binding receptors in the liver.

Stem cell   An unspecialized cell that gives rise to differentiated cells.

Steroid   Any of numerous natural or synthetic compounds containing a 17-carbon 4-ring system, including the sterols and various hormones and glycosides.

T cell   Any of several lymphocytes that differentiate in the thymus, possess highly specific cell-surface antigen receptors, and control the initiation or suppression of cell-mediated and acquired immunity.

T cell receptor (TCR)   The characteristic cell surface protein of T cells that recognizes and binds to human leukocyte antigen molecules and is thereby sensitized to "self" or "nonself" epitopes.

Transgenic animal   An animal into which one or more genes from another species have been incorporated.

Tremor   A trembling or shaking.

Vaccination   The introduction into humans or animals of microorganisms that have been treated to make them harmless for the purpose of inducing the development of immunity.

Virus   Any of a large group of noncellular infective agents that can reproduce only in living cells and that can cause various diseases in humans, animals, or plants.

Vitamin   Any of various organic substances that are essential in the diet, in small amounts act as coenzymes or precursors of coenzymes, and are present in natural foodstuffs.

Index

Understanding Health and Sickness Series
Miriam Bloom, Ph.D., General Editor

Also in this series